T0234002

# Primer on Risk Analysis

## Decision Making Under Uncertainty

### Second Edition

# Primer on Risk Analysis

## Decision Making Under Uncertainty

### Second Edition

Charles Yoe

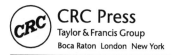

CRC Press
Taylor & Francis Group
Boca Raton  London  New York

CRC Press is an imprint of the
Taylor & Francis Group, an **informa** business

CRC Press
Taylor & Francis Group
6000 Broken Sound Parkway NW, Suite 300
Boca Raton, FL 33487-2742

© 2019 by Taylor & Francis Group, LLC
CRC Press is an imprint of Taylor & Francis Group, an Informa business

No claim to original U.S. Government works

Printed on acid-free paper

International Standard Book Number-13: 978-1-138-31228-9 (Paperback)
978-0-367-07518-7 (Hardback)

### Library of Congress Cataloging-in-Publication Data

Names: Yoe, Charles E., author.
Title: Primer on risk analysis : decision making under uncertainty / Charles Yoe.
Description: Second edition. | Boca Raton : Taylor & Francis, CRC Press, 2019. | Includes bibliographical references.
Identifiers: LCCN 2018044468| ISBN 9781138312289 (pbk. : alk. paper) | ISBN 9780367075187 (hardback : alk. paper) | ISBN 9780429664878 (ePub) | ISBN 9780429662157 (Mobi/Kindle)
Subjects: LCSH: Risk assessment. | Decision making.
Classification: LCC T57.95 .Y62 2019 | DDC 658.15/5--dc23
LC record available at https://lccn.loc.gov/2018044468

**Visit the Taylor & Francis Web site at**
**http://www.taylorandfrancis.com**

**and the CRC Press Web site at**
**http://www.crcpress.com**

*Notre Dame of Maryland University, my employer for the last 30 or so years, is one of those rare institutions that lives its mission. The first sentence in our mission statement is, "Notre Dame of Maryland University educates leaders to transform the world." I believe the science of risk analysis can improve decision making and decision outcomes. I hope this Primer contributes to that mission in some small way.*

# Contents

# Preface

*Principles of Risk Analysis: Decision Making Under Uncertainty* was my passion. It is the extended version of this Primer. Truth be told, the Primer was a pitch I made to try to help convince my publisher to do the Principles. It turned out there was an interest in and a need for a Primer. There are a lot of individuals and communities of practice (CoP) that want to know some basics of risk analysis science. The discipline is evolving and so the Primer is too.

In this second edition, there are two new chapters. The first one addresses enterprise risk management (ERM), one of the fastest growing applications of risk analysis science. ERM has been the entry point to risk analysis for many private sector organizations. You will learn the basics of this unique application there. The second chapter, Decision Making Under Uncertainty, is a practical chapter for risk managers and decision makers who are being tasked with making risk-informed decisions. It has been evident to me, in my consulting practice, that decision makers need some practical advice on how to make risk-informed decisions. This chapter marks a first attempt to provide that advice. Each of the other five chapters has been tweaked and updated.

In this Primer, I have tried to distill the basic principles of risk analysis science in a way that does not depend on any one discipline or application of these principles. The principles found within these pages are as valid for the food safety CoP as the U.S. Environmental Protection Agency, a university, or a private business. It is my sincere hope that users of this Primer will find it valuable for gaining an understanding of risk management, risk assessment, and risk communication, as well as those who will make decisions based on the information generated by these three tasks.

# About the Author

**Charles Yoe** is a professor of economics at Notre Dame of Maryland University and director of its wholly online Master of Science in Risk Management degree program. An independent risk analysis consultant and trainer, he has worked extensively for U.S. and other government agencies as a consultant and risk analyst, his wide range of risk experience includes engineering, international trade, food safety, natural disasters, public works, homeland security, ecosystem restoration, resource development, navigation, planning, and water resources. As a consultant to private industry, his work includes a discrete but wide variety of concerns. He has assisted major government agencies in their transition to enterprise risk management, trained professionals from over 100 countries in risk assessment and risk management, and has conducted customized risk training programs for government agencies and private industry in over two dozen nations. He can be reached at cyoe1@verizon.net.

# chapter one

# The basics

## 1.1   What is risk?

Risk is a measure of the probability and consequence of uncertain future events. It is the chance of an undesirable outcome. That outcome could be a loss due to fire, flood, illness, death, financial setback, or any sort of hazard, or a potential gain that is not realized because a new product did not catch on as hoped, your investment did not produce expected benefits, the ecosystem was not restored, or any sort of opportunity was missed. What usually creates the "chance" is a lack of information about events that have not yet occurred. We lack information because there are facts we do not know, the future is fundamentally uncertain, and because the universe is inherently variable. Let's call all of this "uncertainty" for the moment.

Given the presence of a hazard or an opportunity, there are two important components to a risk: an undesirable outcome or consequence and the chance or probability it will occur. Risk is often described by the simple equation:

$$\text{Risk} = \text{Consequence} \times \text{Probability} \qquad (1.1)$$

Consider this expression a mental model that helps us think about risk rather than an equation that defines it. What this expression is conveying is not so much that this is the manner in which all risks are calculated (they are not) as much as that both of these elements must be present for there to be a real risk. If an event of any consequence has no probability of occurrence, there is no risk. Likewise, if there is no consequence or undesirable outcome, then there is no risk.

A hazard is the thing that causes the potential for an adverse consequence. An opportunity causes the potential for a positive consequence. If a population, an individual, or some asset of interest to us is not exposed to the hazard or opportunity, then there will be no consequence and no risk. The range of possible consequences, loss of life, property damage, financial loss or gain, improved environmental conditions, product success, and the like is vast, but even similar types of consequences can vary in frequency, magnitude, severity, and duration.

It is not likely that many risk professionals would agree with such simple definitions. There are any number of alternative definitions in use or found in the literature. Some purists prefer to define risk entirely in terms of adverse consequences, ignoring the chance of gains that may not be realized. These risks of loss are sometimes called pure risks. Some definitions specify the nature of the consequences. The U.S. Environmental Protection Agency (EPA), for example, "considers risk to be the chance of harmful effects to human health or to ecological systems resulting from exposure to an environmental stressor" (EPA, 2010).

Storms, hurricanes, floods, forest fires, and earthquakes are examples of natural hazards. When humans and human activity are exposed to these hazards, there are risks with consequences that include loss of life, property damage, economic loss, and so on. There are human-made hazards by the scores: tools, weapons, vehicles, chemicals, technology, and activities that can pose risks to life, property, environment, economies, and the like. Health hazards comprise their own category and include pathogens, disease, and all manner of personal health difficulties and accidents that can arise. These risks of adverse consequences are traditional examples of risk.

Less widely accepted as risks, among the risk analysis community's members, are potential gains or rewards. Would anyone say they risk a promotion or an inheritance? Probably not, as this is not the traditional use of the word. Nonetheless, when there is some uncertainty that the gain will be realized, it qualifies as a risk under the definition used here. The International Organization for Standardization defines risk as the effect of uncertainty on an organization's objectives (ISO, 2018). This is clearly broad enough to include uncertain opportunities for gain. Risks of uncertain gain are often called speculative risks.

## THE LANGUAGE IS MESSY

The language of risk is relatively young and still evolving. The seeds of risk analysis are sown across many disciplines and each has found it useful to define the terms of risk analysis in a way that best serves the needs of the parent discipline. The EPA, for example, identifies 19 variations on the meaning of risk in their *Thesaurus of Terms Used in Microbial Risk Assessment*, which eponymously takes a narrow focus on the concept of risk (EPA, 2007).

Frank Knight (1921) is credited with the first modern definition of risk. Kaplan and Garrick (1981) attempted to unify the language with their famous triplet. There is not yet any one universally satisfactory definition of risk nor of many of the other terms used in this book. ISO 31000, for example, offers quite a different lexicon than the one used in this book (ISO, 2018). There is more agreement on the practice of risk analysis than there is on its language.

For those who prefer to think of risks only as adverse consequences, it takes only a small convolution of thought to say that not realizing the gain/promotion/inheritance is the adverse consequence. In any event, loss and uncertain potential gains are considered risks throughout this book. Know that some would prefer to distinguish and separate risks and rewards more carefully.

Thus, we have pure risks, which are losses with no potential gains and no beneficial result, and speculative or opportunity risks, which are generally defined as risks that result in an uncertain degree of gain. They are further distinguished by the fact that pure risk events are beyond the decision maker's control, the results of uncontrollable circumstances, while speculative risks are the result of conscious choices made in decision making. These two types of risks lead to two distinct risk management strategies: risk avoiding and risk taking. Risk managers select options that will enable them to reduce unacceptable levels of pure risk to acceptable or tolerable levels. Risk managers also choose to take risks when they select an alternative course of action to pursue potential gains. So, risk managers function as risk avoiders when they decide how best to reduce the adverse consequences of risk and as risk takers when they decide how best to realize potential gains in the future. Uncertainty makes all of this necessary; there is no risk without uncertainty.

## A FEW PROPOSITIONS ABOUT RISK

- Risk is everywhere
- Some risks are more serious than others
- Zero risk is not an option
- Risk is unavoidable

Therefore, we need risk analysis to:

- Describe these risks (risk assessment)
- Talk about them (risk communication)
- Do something about the unacceptable ones (risk management)

There is very little we do that is risk free, although risks certainly vary in the magnitudes of their consequences and the frequencies of their occurrences. A leaky ballpoint pen is not in the same class of risks as an asteroid five miles in diameter colliding with Earth.

Risk is sometimes confused with safety. In the past, we have tried to provide safety, and getting to safety has been the goal of many public policies. The problem with a notion like safety is that someone must decide what level of chance or what magnitude of consequence is going to be considered safe. That is a fundamentally subjective decision, and subjective decisions rarely satisfy everyone. Risk, by contrast, can be measurable, objective, and based on fixed criteria.

Safety has been defined in a number of legislative and administrative frameworks* as a "reasonable certainty of no harm," a phrase extended in some contexts to include "when used as intended." The very language chosen suggests the uncertain existence of a residual risk, and if there is a residual risk, then safety in any absolute sense is a psychological fiction. In fact, the act of calling something safe is a risk management decision.

An alternative to looking for safety and providing margins of safety is to look objectively for risk. That means we have to be able to objectively describe these risks for ourselves and others. Then, we need to be able to communicate that information to one another. Finally, we need a means of determining when a risk is not acceptable and needs to be avoided or managed to some level we can tolerate. This is basically the risk analysis process.

Because uncertainty gives rise to risk, the essential purpose of risk analysis is to help us make better decisions under conditions of uncertainty. This is done by separating what we know about a decision problem from what we do not know about the problem. We use what we know and intentionally address those things we do not know in a systematic and transparent decision-making process that includes effective assessment, communication, and management of risks.

Many people in many different disciplines figured this all out a while ago. They also articulated these ideas in the language of their own disciplines, and that has given birth to a wonderfully chaotic language of risk. Many of these discipline-based uses of risk analysis have deep enough roots that practitioners are sometimes reluctant to consider other views of this new composite discipline. There may be emerging consensus about some ideas, but there is little or no universal agreement about the language of risk analysis. That makes it difficult for anyone trying to understand the essence of risk analysis to get a clear view of just what this is all about.

Risk analysis is a framework for decision making under uncertainty. It was born spontaneously, if not always simultaneously, in many disciplines. It has evolved by fits and starts rather than by master design. Its practice is a wonderful mess of competing and even, at times, contradictory models. Its language borders on a babel of biblical proportions. And still it has begun to become something we can all recognize.

Many practitioners do not even recognize the term "risk analysis." They would call this framework for decision making under uncertainty "risk management." They could argue, effectively, that it includes risk

---

* The Food Quality Protection Act of 1996 is one such example.

assessment and risk communication. The language of risk is quite messy and not likely to be reconciled any time soon.

This book makes no pretense toward unifying, standardizing, or exemplifying the language, definitions, or models of the science of risk analysis. What it does modestly attempt is to distill the common elements and principles of the many risk tribes and dialects into serviceable definitions and narratives. There is more that unites risk analysis and risk management than divides it. Once grounded in the basic principles of risk analysis, or, if you prefer, risk management, the reader should feel free to venture forth into the applications and concepts of the many communities of practice to use their models and speak their language. Now, with this simple understanding of risk and this caveat in mind, let's consider a few more important questions.

## 1.2   How do we identify a risk?

It is precisely because the language is so messy that it is important to be able to identify a risk clearly. There are five essential steps to a good risk identification process:

- Identify the trigger event.
- Identify the hazard or opportunity for uncertain gain.
- Identify the specific harm or harms that could result from the hazard or opportunity for uncertain gain.
- Specify the sequence of events that is necessary for the hazard or opportunity for uncertain gain to result in the identified harm(s).
- Identify the most significant uncertainties in the preceding steps.

### 1.2.1   Trigger

Something initiates the need for risk identification. It could be a discrete event like a study authorization or a flood, information obtained from stakeholders, the accumulation of scientific knowledge, an intentional search for risks, and the like. It helps to note the event that triggers a specific risk coming to light.

### 1.2.2   Hazard or opportunity

A hazard is anything that is a potential source of harm to a valued asset. Hazards include all natural and anthropogenic events capable of causing adverse effects on people, property, economy, culture, social structure, or environment. Hazards can be readily fit into such categories of hazards as biological, chemical, physical, and radiological agents. Examples of hazardous events include terrorism, infrastructure failure, crimes, fires, hurricanes, wars, explosions, seismic events, hydraulic fracturing, automobile accidents, and so on.

An opportunity is any situation that causes, creates, or presents the potential for an uncertain positive consequence. It is any set of circumstances that presents a good opportunity for progress, advancement, or other desirable gain to a valued asset. The gain may be personal, organizational, communal, societal, national, or global. Opportunities include potential financial gain through new products, ventures, and behaviors, and they also include such things as cost savings, ecosystem improvements, reduced traffic congestion, and so on.

---

**LOSS RISK**

*Trigger*: Congressional authorization
*Hazard*: Aquatic nuisance species (ANS)
*Harm*: Reduced landings of commercial fisheries
*Sequence*: Pathway exists → ANS arrives at pathway → ANS survives passage through pathway → ANS colonizes in commercial fishery waterway → ANS spreads and outcompetes commercial fishery
*Uncertainty*: Arrival time, survival through pathway, will it outcompete

**SPECULATIVE RISK**

*Trigger*: Competition among ports
*Opportunity*: Reduce transportation costs
*Harm*: Reductions not realized
*Sequence*: Harbor improvements → fleet composition does not change → tonnage lost to other ports
*Uncertainty*: Fleet composition, trade patterns, technology changes

---

## 1.2.3   Consequence

Determining the specific harm in a risk situation must precede an assessment of the probability of that harm. Thus, consequence comes before probability in the risk identification task. If one begins with the probability, it is easy to become confused: the probability of what? Once the consequence is identified, it is easier to identify its probability. Analysts must identify the specific harm or harms that can result from a hazard. Likewise, they must identify the disappointing and unwelcomed results that can occur with an opportunity for uncertain gain.

There may be more than one undesirable outcome. If so, identify all the relevant harms to be assessed. Floods for example can result in loss of life, property damage, business loss, and other kinds of harm. Ecosystem restoration could increase habitat, improve water quality, increase ecosystem services, and offer other potential gains.

### 1.2.4    Sequence of events

For each harm identified, the analyst should identify the specific sequence of events that is necessary for the hazard to result in the identified harm or consequence. The likelihood of that precise sequence of events occurring will define the probability of the risk. When there is more than one pathway from the hazard to the harm, each relevant pathway ought to be identified. In a similar fashion, the sequence of events from an opportunity to an undesirable outcome ought to be identified.

### 1.2.5    Uncertainty

The initial identification of a risk is likely to be uncertain. Some consequences, that is, harms, may be uncertain and the sequence of events that leads to them may, likewise, be uncertain. Even when the consequences and their causative events are known, there can be uncertainty about their magnitude, frequency, duration, and the like. It is the analyst's job to identify the most significant uncertainties that attend a risk so that they can be addressed in assessment and management.

This identification process provides clarity about the risk of concern. It is common practice to speak about the risk of acrylamide, the risk of dam failure, the risk of bankruptcy, and so on. This shorthand communication often leads to considerable confusion about the true nature of a risk. For risk managers, assessors, and communicators, it is essential that they are able to clearly and unambiguously identify risks of concern with a process like that above before they revert to shorthand descriptions of risks.

## 1.3    What is risk analysis?

Risk analysis is an emerging science and it is a decision-making paradigm. Terje Aven (2018) makes a powerful argument for risk analysis as a new emerging science. Although it is rapidly developing, it is not yet widely regarded as a science unto itself. As a paradigm, it is capable of producing knowledge about risks and risky activities in the real world. As a science, it also produces knowledge about concepts, theories, frameworks, methods, and the like to understand, assess, communicate, and manage risks. This latter knowledge set makes risk analysis as much a science as statistics is, for example. The risk analysis paradigm presented in this text is frequently referred to as risk management, especially by those who practice enterprise risk management.

**PILLARS OF RISK ANALYSIS SCIENCE**

1. The Scientific Basis
2. Concepts
3. Risk Assessment
4. Risk Perception and Communication
5. Risk Management
6. Solving Real Risk Problems and Issues

**Source: Aven (2018)**

The traditional scientific method is often not applicable for decision making, especially when uncertainties are large and social values are prominent. Risk analysis is a process for decision making under uncertainty that consists of three tasks: risk management, risk assessment, and risk communication, as shown in Figure 1.1. We can think of it as

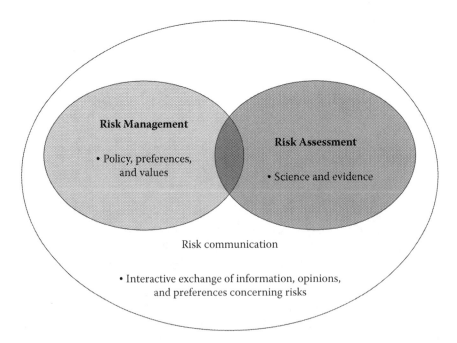

*Figure 1.1* Three tasks of risk analysis.

the process of examining the whole of a risk by assessing the risk and its related relevant uncertainties for the purpose of efficacious management of the risk, facilitated by effective communication about the risk. It is a systematic way of gathering, recording, and evaluating information that can lead to recommendations for a decision or action in response to an identified hazard or opportunity for gain.

Risk analysis for real-world problems is not certain; it is not a solution; it is not static. We may be uncertain about one or more aspects of the consequence of the risk(s) of concern to us or its likelihood of occurring. More troubling, we may be unsure of what to do about the risk or how effective our risk management efforts will be. Risk analysis should address all these things as a paradigm for decision making under conditions of uncertainty. Thus, we draw a distinction between the science of risk analysis that advances the field and the risk analysis paradigm that is applied to real-world problems.

> I speak the dialect of the community of practice (CoP) that raised me in risk. That would be the public sector, with stewardship responsibilities for public health and safety and natural resources. If your CoP prefers to use risk management as the overarching term to organize and label its risk work, I honestly believe you can substitute risk management for risk analysis without doing any significant harm at all to the discipline of risk. Do not let that distinction get in your way of learning. Risk management takes center stage as an organizing concept in the chapter on enterprise risk management.

People tend to not be terribly analytical when making decisions. Human reasoning is fallible. Risk analysis influences our thinking by making it more analytical. This simultaneously limits the "damage" our fallible human reasoning can inadvertently do when making decisions. Risk analysis is a useful and an evolving way to think about and solve risky and uncertain problems. It is "science-based" decision making. This is true in part because the uncertainty is sometimes substantial, but also because risk analysis honors social values. In fact, it is not a stretch to think of risk analysis as the decision-making interface between science and values.

What makes risk analysis a science and a paradigm? That question will be answered in some detail throughout this book. But let's consider a few features that distinguish it.

First, it is based on good science. Scientific facts, evidence, and good analytical techniques are hallmarks of risk analysis. In best practice, risk analysis relies on the best available science. Risk analysis separates what we know (the science) from what we don't know (the uncertainty), and it focuses appropriate attention on what we don't know and how that might affect decision outcomes and, therefore, the decision itself. It aspires to get the right science into the decision process and then to get that science right. The risk assessment task is always based as much as possible on sound evidence, whether that evidence is qualitative or quantitative, known with certainty or shadowed by uncertainty. Done well, risk analysis uses the best available analytical techniques and methods.

Second, risk analysis considers social values. As important as science is, it is not the sole basis for decision making. Social values enter the risk analysis process through the risk management task. Risk analysis incorporates both good science and social values when making decisions under uncertainty.

Third, risk analysis addresses uncertainty explicitly. Few, if any, decisions are ever made with complete information and certainty. Lacking complete information and facing sometimes considerable uncertainty rarely absolves us of the need to make a decision. Risk analysis has evolved explicitly for these kinds of decision problems. It is a paradigm that copes well with soft data and that tolerates ambiguity both in analysis and decision making. Risk assessors address uncertainty in the assessment of risks, risk managers address it in their decision making, and risk communicators convey its significance to interested parties as appropriate.

Fourth, the purpose of this paradigm is to begin to make good decisions by finding and defining the right problem. If the problem is not properly identified, little that follows will aid a successful solution. Risk analysis seeks the needed information from a variety of sources. In the process of doing so, it involves many people in its efforts to identify and resolve that which we do not know about the problem.

Fifth, because of its focus on uncertainty, risk analysis is well suited to continuously improving decisions. As uncertainty is reduced over time and problems are better understood, new and better solutions may come into view. Risk analysis is flexible and can be updated. Every risk management decision is conditional on what is known and what is not known at the time the decision is made. Risk analysis has an eye on uncertainty, and this enables it to deal with a future-focused vision of the next solution as well as the current one. Reducing that which is not yet known about a situation and ever-changing social values ensures that many risk management decisions are part of an evolutionary decision-making process.

Risk analysis provides information to decision makers; it does not make decisions. It is neither a magic bullet nor a black box. The risk analysis paradigm helps establish the balance between the expediency of decision making and having all the information. It does not remove subjectivity and judgment from decision making. If anything, it shines a light on these things and forces us to consider what is not known with certainty.

Risk analysis is defined here as a process with three tasks. These tasks are discussed in considerable detail in subsequent chapters. For now, let us content ourselves with some informal characterizations of these tasks.

## 1.3.1   Risk management

Risk management is a process of problem identification, requesting information, evaluating risks, and initiating action to identify, evaluate, select, implement, monitor, and modify actions taken to alter levels of unacceptable risk to acceptable or tolerable levels. The goals of risk management are often said to include scientifically sound, cost-effective, integrated actions that reduce risks while taking into account economic, environmental, social, cultural, ethical, political, and legal considerations. More informally, risk management is the work one has to do to pose and then answer the following kinds of questions:

1. What is the problem?
2. What information do we need to solve it, that is, what questions do we want risk assessment to answer?
3. What can be done to reduce the impact of the risk described?
4. What can be done to reduce the likelihood of the risk described?
5. What are the trade-offs of the available options?
6. What is the best way to address the described risk?
7. (Once implemented) Is it working?

Risk management is discussed at length in Chapter 3 and a description of enterprise risk management is provided in Chapter 6.

### REWARDS

When the definition of risk is expanded to include uncertain potential gains, it challenges the conventional language. In particular, risk management must include modifying risks as well as mitigating them. Some of the informal questions posed must be altered somewhat.

- What is the opportunity?
- What information do we need to attain it, that is, what questions do we want risk assessment to answer?

- What can be done to increase the positive impact of the opportunity risk described?
- What can be done to increase the likelihood of the desired outcomes?

The other questions remain the same for either risk of loss or opportunity risk.

The alternating emphasis on potential gains could become tedious and cumbersome if constantly continued. Alternative discussions of potential gains will be restricted to only the most critical topics. If you find the language confusing at times for a potential gain, it may help to consider failure to attain the gain as a loss.

### 1.3.2   Risk assessment

Risk assessment is a systematic process for describing the nature, likelihood, and magnitude of risk associated with some substance, situation, action, or event that includes consideration of relevant uncertainties. Risk assessment can be qualitative, quantitative, or a blend (semiquantitative) of both. It can be informally described by posing and answering the following questions that build on the Kaplan and Garrick triplet (1981):

1. What can go wrong?
2. What are the consequences?
3. How can it happen?
4. How likely is it to happen?

### 1.3.3   Risk communication

Risk communication is the open, two-way exchange of information and opinion about risks intended to lead to a better understanding of the risks and better risk management decisions. It provides a forum for the interchange of information with all concerned about the nature of the risks, the risk assessment, and how risks should be managed. Risk communication may be informally characterized by its own set of questions (Chess and Hance, 1994):

1. Why are we communicating?
2. Who are our audiences?
3. What do our audiences want to know?
4. How will we communicate?
5. How will we listen?

6. How will we respond?
7. Who will carry out the plans? When?
8. What problems or barriers have we planned for?
9. Have we succeeded?

### 1.3.4   Risk semantics

Even a brief review of the literature will reveal a staggering range of definitions for these tasks. As with the definitions of risk, the discipline of origin and the nature of the risk have a powerful influence over the words used to define these tasks. However, once the words are distilled to their essence, the ideas represented by the questions above capture the spirit of most definitions in use today. The differences are, in my opinion, more semantic than substantive, but semantics are very important to some people. Any good risk analysis approach will identify hazards and opportunities, characterize the risks, recognize and address uncertainty, summarize conclusions, recommend options, make decisions and document the basis for all recommendations and decisions.

## 1.4   Why do risk analysis?

In a word, "uncertainty" is the reason we do risk analysis. There is very little in life that is risk free, and risk is everywhere. Even in a certain world, decision making may not be a seamless process. We would still argue values, priorities, and trade-offs, for example; but it would be much easier than it is now. In the uncertain world in which we live, the circumstances of our lives, the problems we face, and the evidence we need as well as the outcomes of our decisions are often unknown. We have come to realize the value found in managing, assessing, and communicating about risks to make better decisions and to better inform affected publics and stakeholders about the nature of the risks they face and the steps we take to manage them.

There are also other compelling reasons. Our decision-making processes and approaches to problems used in the past have paid amazing dividends. We have done much to make the world less risky through modern medicine, engineering, finance, environmental management, and the like. Even so, substantial and persistent problems remain. New risks appear all the time. Clearly, as well as our decision processes have served us in the past, they have not been sufficient to rid the world of risks. So, we do risk analysis to intentionally make our lives less risky, to wisely take risks when warranted and, hopefully, to reduce unacceptable risks to levels that we can at least tolerate.

Traditional approaches to decision making have relied on such things as precedent, trial and error, expert opinion, professional judgment, compromise, safety assessment, standards, precaution, inspection, zero tolerance, ignorance, and a host of other somewhat structured decision-making strategies. These traditional approaches have proven insufficient, as recurring problems and unrealized opportunities persist. They have been unable to detect and resolve many current problems. They have been slow to effectively deal with the growing complexity and rapid pace of change in society. Few of these traditional approaches have effectively integrated science and social values in decision making. They do not deal especially well with uncertainty.

Science-based risk analysis activities have been shown to be effective in reducing risks, and they are becoming the standard operating procedure for many public- and private-sector organizations. Risk analysis adds value to decisions by improving the quality of our thinking before a decision is made. Uncertainty is ubiquitous, and every organization develops its own culture of uncertainty. At one extreme, this culture is dominated by risk analysis; at the opposite extreme, we are oblivious to what we do not know. Intentionally considering the relevant uncertainty in a decision problem improves decision making.

One of the principal reasons we do risk analysis is to help provide and ensure a safer living and working environment for people. Risk analysis has also been used extensively to help protect animals, plant life, ecosystems, infrastructure, property, financial assets, and other aspects of modern society. Risk analysis has become essential to economic development. The Technical Barriers to Trade (TBT) and Sanitary Phytosanitary (SPS) Agreements of the World Trade Organization, for example, establish risk assessment as a legitimate means for establishing protective trade practices when the life, health, and safety of a sovereign nation's people are at risk. Risk analysis and risk assessment are being used more and more frequently by domestic and international organizations.

## 1.5   Who does risk analysis?

Many risk analysis practices have been around for centuries. However, it is only in the last half century or so that the practice of risk analysis has started to become more formalized and structured. Government agencies use risk analysis as the basis for regulation, resource allocation, and other risk management decisions. Private industry, sometimes following government's lead and sometimes leading government, is also making more frequent and widespread use of risk analysis, although it may be more common for them to refer to the overarching concept as risk management. To understand who is using risk analysis, it is helpful to begin with a brief history of its evolution.

## 1.5.1    A brief historical perspective on risk analysis

Risk analysis was not possible until we were able to think intentionally about the facts of what can go wrong, how it can happen, its consequences, and the probabilities of those consequences occurring. Anyone who wants to know the history of risk analysis needs to read *Against the Gods: The Remarkable Story of Risk* (Bernstein, 1996). If there is not time to read this book, then read Covello and Mumpower's (1985) *Risk Analysis and Risk Management: An Historical Perspective.* These are simply the best single works of their genres done on the subject. This section owes a great debt to each.

We have always faced problems and have solved them, more or less successfully, since we have walked the planet. The authors cited in the previous paragraph detail this history delightfully. It was the possibility of risk assessment, however, that opened the door for risk analysis, and risk assessment has been made possible by the confluence of many events throughout history. These include the development of probabilistic thinking, which enables us to thoughtfully consider the "chance" dimension of risk and the evolution of science, which enables us to analyze and understand the "undesirable outcomes" that can occur. Our ability to think about and to understand probability and consequences in risk scenarios made risk assessment possible.

The rise of decision sciences, especially in the last century, has enhanced the role of the manager in the analysis of risk. Our growing interest in finding effective ways to deal with uncertainty in the universe has magnified the importance of both the assessment and management tasks. The fact that we still face many old as well as a growing number of new and emerging problems not solved by our old decision-making paradigms has opened the door for risk analysis at this point in time. Growing emphasis on the involvement of the public and stakeholders in public policy decisions has created a role for risk communication. So, let us begin a brief look at the historical development of our ability to think about probability and the development of scientific methods to establish and demonstrate causal links and connections between adverse effects and different types of hazards and activities.

Undoubtedly, risk assessment began when some unknown *Homo sapiens* picked up something, ate it, fell sick, and died. "Don't eat that!" must have been the mental note all those around him made. Risk analysis had begun.

History is filled with scientific footnotes that suggest aspects of risk assessment. The Asipu in 3200 BCE (Covello and Mumpower, 1985) plied the Tigris-Euphrates Valley offering guidance for risky ventures. Centuries later, Hippocrates (460–377 BCE) studied the toxicity of lead. Socrates (469–399 BCE) experienced the risks of hemlock, and Aristotle (384–322 BCE) knew that fumes from charcoal could be dangerous. Pliny (23–79 CE) and Galen (131–201 CE) explored the toxicity of mercury in their medical studies. The point being, we humans have long been engaged with aspects of risk, especially identifying those things that can do us harm.

Fast forward to the later Renaissance period in Europe where gambling, always a popular pastime, piqued an interest in the more formal study of probability. If anyone succeeded in figuring out the odds of various games of chance, it was not documented until Girolamo Cardano (1500–1571) wrote *Liber de Ludo Aleae* (Book on Games of Chance). This is one of the earliest works to explore statistical principles of probability. His book, which focused on chance, is the first to express chance as a fraction. Odds began to appear soon after.

Blaise Pascal's (1623–1662) wager is broadly considered to be one of the first examples of decision science. Pascal undertook the age-old question of God's existence: God is, or God is not? Which way should we incline, and how shall we live our lives? Considering two states of the world (God is, God is not) and two alternative behaviors (live as a Christian, live as a pagan), Pascal used probability and concluded that the expected value of being a Christian outweighed the expected value of paganism.

The use of basic statistics is also relatively new to humans. John Graunt (1620–1674) undertook a study of births and deaths in seventeenth-century London to learn how many people may be available for military service. He used raw data in new ways, including sampling and statistical inference, that formed the basis for modern statistics. He published his famous life expectancy tables in 1662 and changed data analysis forever.

Risk management made a formal appearance in Edward Lloyd's 1687 London coffeehouse. By 1696, *Lloyd's List* of ship arrivals and departures along with conditions abroad and at sea was a risk management standard for everyone in the British maritime industry. Ships' captains compared notes on hazards in one corner of the coffeehouse and it grew into the headquarters for marine underwriters, a precursor of the modern insurance industry. Flower and Jones (1974) report that London's insurance industry would help protect you from house-breaking, highway robbery, death by gin-drinking, death of horses, and would provide assurance of female chastity—no doubt the great risks of the day!

Jacob Bernoulli (1654–1705) began to integrate ideas about information and evidence into the growing body of thought on probabilities. He noted we rarely know a probability before an event (a priori) but can often estimate a probability after an event (a posteriori). This, he noted, implies changing degrees of belief as more information is compiled; so, the past is only part of reality. Thomas Bayes (1701–1761) extended this work and wrote of using new information to revise probabilities based on old information. The world was beginning to discover tools and to think that perhaps uncertainty can be measured and variability described. Many others, Laplace, Chebyshev, Markov, von Mises, and Kolmogorov, to name a few, followed, and the quantitative universe was gradually being revealed.

Meanwhile, our knowledge of disease and our powers of scientific observation were also making great leaps. Edward Jenner (1749–1823) observed that milkmaids got cowpox but not smallpox. John Snow (1813–1858) figured out that cholera was transmitted by contaminated water, by studying what today we might call a GIS (geographic information system) map of a cholera outbreak. The microscopic world and its risks to health were beginning to come into focus.

The Industrial Revolution marked a change in the public sector's role in the management of risks. Concerns about occupational disease and the need to protect workers and the public from toxic chemicals gave rise to the field of public health. Toxicology was one of many emerging sciences, and the idea of a no observed adverse effects level (NOAEL) was born in the twentieth century. This is the dose of a chemical at which there are no statistically or biologically significant increases in the frequency or severity of adverse effects between the exposed population and its appropriate control. This was clearly a firm step in the direction of risk analysis, combining science with a value judgment.

Early efforts to determine a safe level of exposure to chemicals were based on laboratory animal tests to establish a NOAEL. To leap the uncertain hurdles of extrapolating from animals to humans and from the high doses of a chemical given to animals to the low doses to which humans were exposed, the scientific community approximated a safe level by dividing the NOAEL by an uncertainty or safety factor to establish the acceptable daily intake (ADI):

$$ADI = NOAEL/uncertainty\ factor \qquad (1.2)$$

In the 1950s, the U.S. Food and Drug Administration (FDA) used a factor $= 100$ to account for the uncertainty.

More formal notions of risk were finding their way into the public-sector mentality. The Delaney Clause was a 1958 amendment to the Food, Drug, and Cosmetic Act of 1938 that was an effort to protect the public from carcinogens in food. It is often cited as an effort to establish a zero tolerance for policy purposes. When scientific methods were a bit cruder than they are now, it was easier to equate an inability to detect a hazard with a notion of zero risk.

As science improved, it became clear that zero risk was not a policy option, and the notion of de minimis risk took root. A de minimis risk is a risk so low as to be effectively treated as negligible. Mantel and Bryan (1961) suggested that anything that increases the lifetime risk of cancer by less than 1 in 100 million was negligible. The FDA later relaxed this to 1 in 1 million. The EPA proposed to adopt a uniform "negligible risk" policy for all carcinogenic residues in food in 1988. The Occupational Safety and Health Administration (OSHA) regulated all carcinogens in the workplace to the lowest level feasible. The point to be taken for our purposes is that society was beginning to get used to the idea that we would have to live with some nonzero level of risk.

Risk assessment per se began with radiation biology in the middle of the twentieth century. The Japanese survivors of World War II atomic bomb blasts made the dangers of radiation eminently clear. This new technology raised concerns about how the incidence of human cancer is influenced by exposure to small doses of radiation.

The National Academies of Science (NAS) in the United States struggled with this radiation question, and the first formal risk assessment, "Reactor Safety Study: An Assessment of Accident Risks in U.S. Commercial Nuclear Power Plants," NUREG 75/014, better known as the Rasmussen Report, was prepared for the Nuclear Regulatory Commission (Nuclear Regulatory Commission, 1975). This was, among other things, a study of core meltdowns at nuclear power plants that used a no-threshold model to estimate cancer deaths following a nuclear reactor accident.

## NATIONAL FLOOD PROGRAM

Risk analysis was creeping into the public consciousness in a number of ways, although no one called it by that name at the time. In 1936, the U.S. government passed the Flood Control Act of 1936, which established a national flood control program. This program assesses, communicates, and manages risk. Following hurricanes Katrina and Rita, the U.S. Army Corps of Engineers renamed this program Flood Risk Management.

Government agencies eventually began doing risk assessment routinely, and the early pioneers of risk assessment describe a rather ad hoc process. In the 1980s, the National Research Council was asked to determine whether organizational and procedural reforms could improve the performance and use of risk assessment in the federal government. In 1983, they published their response, *Risk Assessment in the Federal Government: Managing the Process*, better known as "the Red Book" because of its cover (National Research Council, 1983). This is one of the seminal publications in risk assessment and it identified the four steps of risk assessment as:

1. Hazard identification
2. Dose-response assessment
3. Exposure assessment
4. Risk characterization.

   This has been the foundation model for risk assessment that has been modified and evolved many times since.

   Risk assessment came before the U.S. Supreme Court in two cases during the Carter administration. The Industrial Union Department, AFL-CIO v. American Petroleum Institute, 448 U.S. 607 (1980) case considered whether quantitative cancer risk assessments could be used in policy making. One federal agency, OSHA, said no, while the EPA and FDA said yes. The majority opinion established that risk assessment is feasible and that OSHA must do one before taking rule-making action to reduce or eliminate the benzene risk. Later, in the American Textile Manufacturers Institute v. Donovan, 452 U.S. 490 (1981) case, the Supreme Court reaffirmed the Benzene case finding and added that safe does not mean zero risk. With this last hurdle cleared, risk assessment moved more confidently into the government's policy arena.

   Internationally, risk assessment was also growing in credibility. The General Agreement on Tariffs and Trade's (GATT) Uruguay Round on multilateral trade negotiations (1986–1994) was instrumental in the global spread of risk analysis. Specifically, two agreements—on Sanitary and Phytosanitary Measures (SPS) and on Technical Barriers to Trade (TBT)— paved the way for risk assessment in the World Trade Organization (WTO).

## THREE SISTERS

The SPS agreement has influenced the international standards of the *Codex Alimentarius* (for food), the World Organization for Animal Health (OIE), and the International Plant Protection Convention (IPPC) all of whom have adopted risk analysis principles for their procedures.

   The SPS agreement (1995) recognizes the right of governments to protect the health of their people from hazards that may be introduced with imported food by imposing sanitary measures, even if this meant trade restrictions. The agreement obliges governments to base such sanitary measures on risk assessment to prevent disguised trade protection measures.

   Following the lead of the WTO, many regional trade agreements, including the North American Free Trade Agreement (NAFTA), incorporate risk analysis principles into their agreements. Both the Food Agricultural Organization (FAO) and the World Health Organization (WHO), two United Nations agencies, lend extensive support to the use of risk analysis principles globally.

The Committee of Sponsoring Organizations of the Treadway Commission (COSO) published its "Enterprise Risk Management-Integrated Framework" in 2004. It defined enterprise risk management (ERM) as a "... process, effected by an entity's board of directors, management, and other personnel, applied in strategy setting and across the enterprise, designed to identify potential events that may affect the entity, and manage risk to be within its risk appetite, to provide reasonable assurance regarding the achievement of entity objectives." The International Organization for Standardization undertook an effort to write a new global guideline for the definition and practice of risk management internationally. That guideline "Risk Management-Principles and Guidelines" was completed and released in 2009 (ISO 31000) it was updated in 2018.

In recent years, many nations have begun to make extensive use of risk analysis in their regulatory and other government functions. Risk analysis is now well established in both the private and public sectors around the world.

## 1.5.2   Government agencies

Government agencies are widely adopting risk analysis principles to varying extents and with varying vocabularies. Some agencies have begun to redefine their missions and modes of operation in terms of risk analysis principles. Risk analysis has become their modus operandi. Other agencies have added risk analysis principles to their existing methodologies and tools for accomplishing their mission (see accompanying text box). *Risk-informed decision making* is a term of art often used to describe the use of risk analysis in some government agencies. States and local governments are adopting risk analysis approaches at varying rates. Natural and environmental resource agencies as well as public health and public safety agencies tend to be the first to adapt risk analysis principles at the nonfederal levels of government.

Internationally, risk analysis has proliferated in some communities of practice. Food safety, animal health, plant protection, engineering, and the environment are some of the areas in which other national governments are likely to have established the practice of risk analysis. The global economic recession that began in 2008 has propelled economic and financial regulatory agencies to move more aggressively toward risk analysis, in the form of ERM.

## SELECTED U.S. AGENCIES USING SOME
## RISK ANALYSIS PRINCIPLES

Animal and Plant Health
 Inspection Service
 http://www.aphis.usda.gov/

Bureau of Economic Analysis (BEA)
 http://www.bea.gov/

Bureau of Reclamation
 http://www.usbr.gov/

Centers for Disease Control and
 Prevention (CDC)
 http://www.cdc.gov/

Coast Guard
 http://www.uscg.mil/

Congressional Budget Office (CBO)
 http://www.cbo.gov/

Consumer Product Safety
 Commission (CPSC)
 http://www.cpsc.gov/

Corps of Engineers
 http://www.usace.army.mil/

Customs and Border Protection
 http://www.cbp.gov/

Defense Advanced Research
 Projects Agency (DARPA)
 http://www.nsf.gov/

Department of Defense (DOD)
 http://www.defenselink.mil/

Department of Energy (DOE)
 http://www.energy.gov/

Department of Homeland Security
 (DHS)
 http://www.dhs.gov

Director of National Intelligence
 http://www.dni.gov

Economic Research Service
 http://www.ers.usda.gov/

Endangered Species Committee
 http://endangered.fws.gov/

Environmental Protection Agency
 (EPA)
 http://www.epa.gov/

Federal Aviation Administration
 (FAA)
 http://www.faa.gov/

Federal Bureau of Investigation
 (FBI)
 http://www.fbi.gov/

Fish and Wildlife Service
 http://www.fws.gov/

Food and Drug Administration
 (FDA)
 http://www.fda.gov/

Food Safety and Inspection Service
 http://www.fsis.usda.gov/

Foreign Agricultural Service
 http://www.fas.usda.gov/

Forest Service
 http://www.fs.fed.us/

Geological Survey (USGS)
 http://www.usgs.gov/

Government Accountability Office
 (GAO)
 http://www.gao.gov/

National Aeronautics and Space
 Administration (NASA)
 http://www.nasa.gov/

National Marine Fisheries
 http://www.nmfs.noaa.gov/

National Oceanic and Atmospheric
 Administration (NOAA)
 http://www.noaa.gov/

National Park Service
 http://www.nps.gov/

National Science Foundation
 http://www.nsf.gov/

National Security Agency (NSA)
http://www.nsa.gov/
National Transportation Safety
Board
http://www.ntsb.gov/
National War College
http://www.ndu.edu/nwc/
index.htm
National Weather Service
http://www.nws.noaa.gov/
Natural Resources Conservation
Service
http://www.nrcs.usda.gov/
Nuclear Regulatory Commission
http://www.nrc.gov/
Oak Ridge National Laboratory
http://www.oro.doe.gov/
Occupational Safety & Health
Administration (OSHA)
http://www.osha.gov/

Office of Management and Budget
(OMB)
http://www.whitehouse.gov/
omb/
Office of Science and Technology
Policy
http://www.ostp.gov/
Risk Management Agency
(Agriculture Department)
http://www.rma.usda.gov/
Securities and Exchange
Commission (SEC)
http://www.sec.gov/
Superfund Basic Research Program
http://www.niehs.nih.gov/
research/supported/sbrp/
Tennessee Valley Authority
http://www.tva.gov/

In 2016, the U.S. Office of Management and Budget Circular No. A-123, *Management's Responsibility for Enterprise Risk Management and Internal Control* established the requirement for U.S. Government agencies to implement an ERM capability in order to improve mission delivery, reduce costs, and focus corrective actions toward key risks.

## 1.5.3   Private sector

The insurance industry may represent the oldest and most explicit application of risk management in the private sector. As early as 1955, Dr. Wayne Snider, University of Pennsylvania, suggested "the professional insurance manager should be a risk manager." By 1966, the Insurance Institute of America had created a credentialed position called "Associate in Risk Management." In 1975, the American Society of Insurance Management changed its name to the Risk and Insurance Management Society (RIMS). In 1986, the Institute for Risk Management in London began a program of continuing education that looked at risk management in all its aspects. GE Capital used the title "Chief Risk Officer" to describe an organizational function to manage all aspects of risk that same year.

During the 1990s, several national standards began advocating that businesses should manage all risks as a portfolio across the enterprise. COSO's "Enterprise Risk Management-Integrated Framework" was a significant step forward. By the time ISO 31000 was published in 2009, the private sector had two popular models of risk management to follow. Both of these models include the three risk analysis tasks of risk management, risk assessment, and risk communication, to varying extents. The private financial sector has also been an innovator in risk-related areas. Security has taken on a growing number of risk applications as technology has expanded the notion of and need for risk analysis. Academia has also embraced risk management in significant numbers.

Risk management spread from the insurance and financial sectors to other safety-oriented professions and businesses like engineering, construction, and manufacturing, where safety assessments have long been a part of the industry. From there it has been a short leap to every kind of private entity. Organizations in all industries have now begun a more explicit consideration of risk.

A conspicuous example of this is found in the food industry, where all links in the food chain have been devoting increased attention to food-safety risk analysis. The medical community is also increasingly involved with risk reduction. Formal risk analysis/risk management has been penetrating the private sector in increasingly large numbers. ISO 31000 marks a landmark effort to standardize many risk management notions for industry. As public policies increasingly reflect the influence of risk analysis, it is inevitable that the private-sector interest will continue to grow. A 2016 survey of over 300 U.S.-based executives (Deloitte, 2017) identified the following top-rated risk management successes in private industry (% of respondents):

- Avoided major compliance failures (44%)
- Expanded our senior leadership team's participation in setting risk management priorities (42%)
- Have become more agile through risk management (36%)
- Identified and acted on an important opportunity for a new product or line of business (31%)
- Avoided a major reputational damage (31%)
- Improved risk management by implementing new methods/ technologies (28%)
- Avoided a major potential financial loss (21%)
- Substantially improved relationships with one or more customers (19%)

With these kinds of results, the spread of risk management is inevitable.

## 1.6   When should we do risk analysis?

Risk analysis is for organizations that make decisions under conditions of uncertainty. Figure 1.2 provides a schematic illustration of the kinds of decision contexts where risk analysis adds the most value to decision making. This value depends on how much uncertainty the organization faces and the consequences of making a wrong decision.

In the lower-right quadrant, there is little uncertainty and the consequences of being wrong are minor. This kind of decision making does not require risk analysis. Any convenient means of decision making will do here.

When there is a lot of uncertainty but the consequences of an incorrect decision are minor, it would be sufficient to do a modest level of risk analysis. This may entail little more than sifting through the uncertainty to assure decision makers that the decision and its outcome are not especially sensitive to the uncertainties. In some instances, it may be sufficient to establish that one or the other factors of the "consequence × probability" product is sufficiently small as to render the relevant risks acceptable.

When the consequences of making a wrong decision rise, so does the value of risk analysis. In an environment with relatively less uncertainty but with serious consequences for wrong decisions, risk analysis is valuable as a routine method for decision making. As the uncertainty grows in extent, risk analysis becomes the most valuable, and more-extensive efforts may be warranted.

Some organizations would be wise to always be doing risk analysis. In fact, a slowly growing number of organizations think of themselves as risk

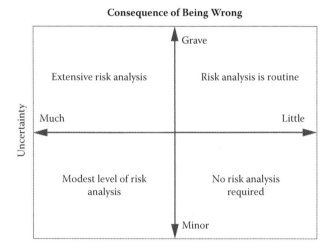

**Figure 1.2** When to use risk analysis.

analysis or risk management organizations, meaning that what they do as an organization is manage risks, assess risks, and communicate about risks. Others use risk analysis as a framework, tool, or methodology for specific situations. Stewards of the public trust would be well advised to use risk analysis for decision making.

Risk analysis, as a way of doing business, is especially useful for organizations that have some or all of the following elements of decision making in common (adapted from National Research Council, 2009):

- A desire to use the best scientific methods and evidence in informing decisions.
- Uncertainty that limits the ability to characterize both the magnitude of the problem and the corresponding benefits of proposed risk management options.
- A need for timeliness in decision making that precludes resolving important uncertainties before decisions are required.
- The presence of some sort of trade-off among disparate values in decision making.
- The reality that, because of the inherent complexity of the systems being managed and the sometimes-long-term implications of many risk management decisions, there may be little or no short-term feedback as to whether the desired outcome has been achieved by the decisions.

Every organization has its own unique reality. They have a history, a mission, personnel, resources, policies, procedures, and their own way of doing things. If you drop risk analysis science down into any organization, the context of that organization is going to affect the way the risk analysis paradigm is going to look and work. For example, there is no agreement on what applied risk science is even called, much less agreement on any one risk analysis model to be followed by the U.S. government agencies mentioned previously. In fact, it is probably fair to say that risk analysis looks different in every organization that uses it.

## WHAT IS IT CALLED?

The EPA favors risk assessment. The FDA and Food Safety Inspection Service tend to use risk analysis. The DoD leans toward integrated risk management, while the U.S. Army Corps of Engineers favors risk-informed decision making.

Take the FDA as an example. Risk analysis is vigorously pursued in several of its Centers including the Centers for Food Safety and Applied

Nutrition, Veterinary Medicine, Devices and Radiological Health, and Drug Evaluation and Research. Each of these defines the terms of risk analysis differently and applies the concepts in different ways and to varying extents. They have developed their own risk-related tools and techniques. This is a strength of the paradigm. It is a remarkably flexible and robust way to think about and to solve problems, so be assured there is no one best way to practice risk analysis.

## 1.7    Organization of this book

This book provides an introduction to the principle tasks of risk analysis science. There are hundreds of very good books already in print devoted to some aspect of risk. Most tend to focus, relatively quickly, on a rather narrow aspect or practice of the discipline. Many are written from a particular disciplinary or topical background, such as engineering, finance, environment, public health, food safety, water resources, and so on. This book avoids a narrow focus on any one field in favor of distilling principles, integrating topics, and stressing the application of the principles in a generic fashion. In particular, it focuses on the most basic principles of the risk analysis paradigm, that is, risk, uncertainty, risk management, risk assessment, and risk communication.

Like good risk analysis, this book proceeds in an iterative fashion. Each of the next four chapters unpacks and explains important concepts introduced in this chapter. Chapter 2 takes up the notion of uncertainty in more detail. Uncertainty is the primary reason for risk analysis and its pervasiveness has caused the use of risk analysis to spread quickly in recent years. It is important for risk managers, risk assessors, and risk communicators to have a sound and common understanding of uncertainty.

Chapter 3 develops the risk management component of risk analysis and the job of the risk manager. In best practice, every risk analysis task begins and ends with risk management. The tasks of risk management are presented in a generic fashion, free from any particular preexisting risk management model. Chapter 4 unpacks the risk assessment component. This is where the analytical work gets done in any risk analysis activity. As with the risk management chapter, the risk assessment tasks are presented free of any specific model. Chapter 5 explores the risk communication component in greater detail. The generic tasks of both the internal and external risk communication responsibilities are presented. These three chapters together describe the risk analysis paradigm.

If you are new to the world of risk, it is possible that the continuing spread of ERM has sparked that interest. ERM has been adopted by a great many private sector organizations, a growing number of nongovernmental organizations (NGO), and more than a few government organizations around the world. It is significantly increasing the footprint of risk analysis. ERM tends to avoid the use of the term "risk analysis" instead using risk management as the overarching term for this risk paradigm. Chapter 6 provides an essential introduction to ERM simply because any primer would be deficient without it.

The final chapter, Chapter 7, reverts back to the fundamental reason for the rise of risk analysis science. The unique value of risk analysis science is that it relies on evidence and a careful and useful characterization of instrumental uncertainty to improve decision making under uncertainty. A practical approach for making decisions under uncertainty is offered in this last chapter, for if risk analysis science does not improve decisions and decision outcomes then it will have failed to reach its fullest potential.

## 1.8   Summary and look forward

Risk is the chance of an undesirable outcome. That outcome may be a loss or the failure to attain a favorable situation. In a certain world, there is no risk because every outcome is known in advance. It is uncertainty that gives rise to risk.

Safety is a subjective judgment, while risk analysis is, in principle, an objective search for the risks in any given situation. Risk analysis is the framework or, if you prefer, the science used to manage, measure, and talk about risk. It has three components: risk management, risk assessment, and risk communication. Risk analysis is now possible because of the confluence of many scientific developments. Its use in the United States and internationally is growing steadily, and applications are found in a wide variety of fields.

The language of risk analysis is evolving. It would be comforting to think that it is evolving toward some consensus definitions and a common terminology. That is not yet the case, and this book makes no attempt to resolve the language differences. What it does do is attempt to distill the principles common to the many different dialects of risk that are spoken in the fields of applied risk analysis. There is a growing tendency among some in both the public and private sectors to refer to the risk analysis paradigm as risk management. This text will use risk analysis to represent the emerging science and to describe the use of risk analysis science as applied to real-world problems. Do not let that semantic debate get in the way of your understanding. Use the term you prefer.

The next chapter gets to the root cause of risk analysis, that is, uncertainty. A primary role of the risk analyst is to separate what we know from what we do not know and then to deal honestly, intentionally, and effectively with those things we do not know. The job of the risk analyst is to be an honest broker of information in decision making. Knowledge uncertainty and natural variability, two fundamental concepts essential to understanding risk analysis, are the focus of Chapter 2.

## References

Aven, T. 2018. An emerging new risk analysis science: Foundations and implications. *Risk Analysis* 38 (5): 876–888.

Bernstein, P. L. 1996. *Against the gods: The remarkable story of risk.* New York: John Wiley & Sons.

Chess, C., and B. J. Hance. 1994. *Communicating with the public: Ten questions environmental managers should ask.* New Brunswick, NJ: Center for Environmental Communication.

Covello, V. T., and J. Mumpower. 1985. Risk analysis and risk management: An historical perspective. *Risk Analysis* 5 (2): 103–120.

Deloitte Risk and Financial Advisory. 2017. *2017 Risk management survey: Shift risk strategies, accelerate performance.* https://www.deloitte.com/us/en/pages/risk/articles/fortune-risk-management-survey.html?id=us:2ps:3bi:risk:en g:adv:112817:na:na:VnBqbWnj:1081889462:76690972547584:bb:Advisory:Fort une_Survey_BMM:nb (accessed April 1, 2018).

Environmental Protection Agency (EPA). 2007. *Thesaurus of terms used in microbial risk assessment.* https://ofmpub.epa.gov/sor_internet/registry/termreg/searchandretrieve/termsandacronyms/search.do?search=&term=risk&ma tchCriteria=Exact&checkedAcronym=true&checkedTerm=true&hasDefini tions=false (accessed October 5, 2018).

Environmental Protection Agency (EPA). 2010. *About risk assessment.* https://www.epa.gov/risk/about-risk-assessment (accessed October 5, 2018).

Flower, R., and M. W. Jones. 1974. *Lloyd's of London: An illustrated history.* Newton Abbot, UK: David and Charles.

International Organization of Standardization (ISO). 2018. *ISO 31000, risk management-guidelines.* Geneva, Switzerland: International Organization of Standardization.

Kaplan, S., and B. J. Garrick. 1981. On the quantitative definition of risk. *Risk Analysis* 1 (1).

Knight, F. H. 1921. *Risk, uncertainty and profit.* Chicago: University of Chicago Press.

Mantel, N., and W. R. Bryan. 1961. Safety testing of carcinogenic agents. *Journal of the National Cancer Institute* 27: 455–470.

National Research Council. 1983. Committee on the Institutional Means for Assessment of Risks to Public Health. *Risk assessment in the federal government: Managing the process.* Washington, DC: National Academies Press.

National Research Council. 2009. Committee on Improving Risk Analysis Approaches Used by the U.S. *EPA. Advancing risk assessment 2009.* Washington, DC: National Academies Press.

Nuclear Regulatory Commission. 1975. *Reactor safety study: An assessment of accident risks in U.S. commercial nuclear power plants.* Washington, DC: Nuclear Regulatory Commission.

# chapter two

# Uncertainty

## 2.1  Introduction

Because risk analysis focuses on decision making under uncertainty, it is important to understand what uncertainty is. At the most basic level, when we are not sure, then we are uncertain. Uncertainty arises at two fundamentally different levels. First, there is the macro-level of uncertainty. We all make decisions in a changing and uncertain decision environment. This means the systems, processes, social values, ways forward, and outcomes of concern to us may be uncertain. Second, there is the micro-level of uncertainty. This is the uncertainty that pertains to specific decision contexts and their relevant knowledge, data, and models. These latter uncertainties receive most of the attention in risk assessment.

If there was no uncertainty about facts, there would be no question about whether or when a loss would occur and how big it would be. Likewise, we would always know how an opportunity would turn out. Even so, uncertainty about what we should do in the face of these situations would still arise because of differing values. Uncertainty is the reason for risk analysis. Risk assessors have to understand uncertainty because they are, in a sense, the first responders to uncertainty. It is the assessors who identify data gaps, holes in our theories, shortcomings of our models, incompleteness in our scenarios, and ignorance about some quantities and variability in others. It is an important part of the risk assessor's* job to address the uncertainty in individual assessment inputs.

Think of the assessor's job as separating what we know from what we do not know about a decision problem context and then being intentional about assessing the significance of the things we do not know for decision making. There are usually things we know with certainty. We can measure distances, count dollars, and we know atomic structures of chemicals; our physical world is loaded with facts. But every decision problem comes with a "pile" of things we do not know. The risk assessor, along with the risk manager, has to identify that pile and what is in it.

---

* The possessive case used for risk assessors and risk managers will always be in the singular form for the sake of simplicity. It should be understood, however, that both can be multiple in numbers at times.

It is the risk manager's job to decide how to handle the uncertainty that remains in decision making. Measures of decision criteria may be uncertain, the outcome of a risk management option may be unknown. Addressing these uncertainty issues is the risk manager's responsibility. There may also be uncertainty that arises with the risk management task. Even when all the decision criteria are clear, the risk manager may not know what to do because of conflicting values. This uncertainty also belongs to the risk manager. Risk managers need to understand uncertainty because they are the final arbiters of it in the decision-making process.

The risk communicator has the responsibility of understanding the uncertainty and its relevance for decision making so that they can explain it and its significance to others. That task requires risk communicators to understand input, output, and outcome uncertainty well enough to make it understandable by diverse audiences among the public and stakeholders interested in a risk management decision.

There is another important distinction to make about things that are uncertain. Uncertainty is relevant if it could impact a decision in at least a subtle way. Relevant uncertainty may make one option less appealing than another or it might make a particular stakeholder uneasy. Relevant uncertainty can be categorized as instrumental or noninstrumental. The ability to distinguish between the two is essential to both good risk assessment and good risk management. Instrumental uncertainty can alter the decision that is made or the outcome of that decision. Noninstrumental uncertainty refers to uncertainty that would not alter a decision if it was reduced. Noninstrumental holes in our data or gaps in information may be relevant in some way, but they would not affect the decision to be made if they were filled. Good risk assessors and risk managers are able to focus on identifying, reducing, or otherwise characterizing the instrumental uncertainty encountered in decision making.

This chapter focuses, in a conceptual way, on the pile of things we do not know and specifically on the instrumental uncertainty in that pile of things. In order to know how best to address the "things" we do not know, the assessor must first understand the nature of those things in the pile of unknowns (see Figure 2.1). The original pile of unknowns, or uncertainty, is then sorted into two distinct sources of not knowing: natural variability and knowledge uncertainty. Natural variability generally refers to empirical quantities. Knowledge uncertainty is divided into three main piles: scenarios and theory, models, and quantities. The quantities, in their turn, are separated into types of quantities first proposed by Morgan and Henrion (1990). This conceptual sorting activity enables us to choose most appropriately from the various tools, techniques, and methodologies available for addressing uncertainty in the assessment and management tasks.

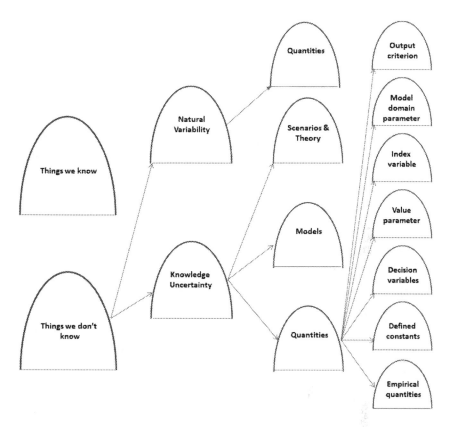

*Figure 2.1* Separating what we know from what we do not know and sorting out the unknowns.

This chapter begins by considering the macro-level of uncertainty that is sometimes overlooked in risk analysis. Then it focuses on the micro-level uncertainty issues that occupy so much of the risk assessor's concerns. At that point in the chapter, we will reengage the structure shown in Figure 2.1.

An important distinction will be drawn between knowledge uncertainty and natural variability, and the many piles illustrated in Figure 2.1 will be explored and discussed. The causes of uncertainty in empirical quantities are considered to round out the discussion of uncertainty as depicted in the figure.

Before beginning, we offer an important clarification of the language. People often speak of uncertain values, and this is, strictly speaking, not correct. The values themselves are not uncertain; it is the assessor and the manager who are uncertain about what a factual value is or what a value that reflects a preference should be. Even so, this text will join in the use of that terminology to avoid the repeated verbosity of explaining that these are values people are uncertain about.

## 2.2   Uncertainty from 75,000 feet

Uncertainty is an emerging constant in modern decision making. We all operate in an uncertain environment. Growing social complexity and an increasingly rapid pace of change are normal parts of the decision-making landscape, and they contribute a great deal to the uncertain environment in which we operate. Risk analysis offers a viable alternative to clinging to a deterministic style of decision making in this uncertain environment.

The world grows more complex. Think of complexity, as used here, in a social sense. It refers to such things as the size of a society, the number of its parts, the distinctiveness of those parts, their interconnectedness, the variety of specialized social roles that it incorporates, the number of distinct social personalities present, and the variety of mechanisms for organizing these into a coherent, functioning whole. Augmenting any of these dimensions increases the complexity of a society (Tainter, 1996). The level of complexity in our social, economic, and technological systems is increasing to a point that is too turbulent and rapidly changing to be wholly understood or predicted by human beings.

### TOP FIVE GLOBAL RISKS

| In terms of likelihood | In terms of impact |
|---|---|
| 1. Extreme weather events | 1. Weapons of mass destruction |
| 2. Natural disasters | 2. Extreme weather events |
| 3. Cyberattacks | 3. Natural disasters |
| 4. Data fraud of thefts | 4. Failure of climate-change |
| 5. Failure of climate-change mitigation and adaptation | mitigation and adaptation |
| | 5. Water crises |

**Source: The Global Risks Report 2018**

For over 99% of human history, we lived as low-density foragers or farmers in egalitarian communities of no more than a few dozen persons and even fewer distinct social roles. In the twenty-first century, we live in societies with millions of different roles and personalities. Our social systems grow so complex as to defy understanding. Consequently, our systems of problem solving have grown more complex.

We face an increasingly rapid pace of change in almost every arena. Scientific breakthroughs make things that once were impossible to conceive commonplace. Much of this change is driven by rapid advances in technology. For example, the risk of conflict is exacerbated by weaponized robotics and artificial intelligence. Cyberspace is an entirely new domain for conflict. Technology changes social values and beliefs as well as the way we live and work. The ways we communicate have changed forever and continue to change in ways that are difficult to forecast. Change is too rapid and at times too unsettled to be wholly understood or predicted.

Social, economic, and technological connectivity around the globe accelerates at a dizzying pace. Social movements are often global in their pervasiveness. We are increasingly a global economy. Fashions are designed in New York and approved in London, patterns are cut in Hong Kong, clothes are made in Taiwan and shipped in containers on vessels that call around the world, and then the clothes are sold across Europe and North America. Computer viruses spread in hours; human viruses spread in weeks. We are indelibly connected.

With government deficits and debts rising in the more established economies of the world, there is relentless pressure on costs in all public decision making. Patterns of competition are becoming unpredictable. It is getting harder and harder to understand and anticipate who the competition is for a job, for U.S. grain, for land use, and so on. For businesses and government agencies alike, customer/client profiles are changing rapidly and unpredictably. We see quickly increasing and diversified customer demands. There is a growing role for one-of-a-kind services and production, and rapid sequences of new tasks in business and government are becoming more routine. A media explosion is just one of the consequences of an increase in the number and speed of communication channels. Big data is transforming the ways that businesses operate.

As a result of these and other changes, we have entered a world where irreversible consequences, unlimited in time and space, are now possible. This is, or should be, extremely important to risk managers in both the public and private sectors. Decades after the accident at Chernobyl, some of its victims haven't even been born yet. Some of the wicked problems* risk managers face can have a long latency period. Many of the United States' landscape-scale ecosystem restoration problems—like those in the Florida Everglades, Coastal Louisiana, and the Columbia River basin—as well as such global concerns as greenhouse gases, climate change, and sea level rise provide clear examples of problems that took decades to emerge and

---

* Wicked problems are complex problems that lack right and wrong solutions. Instead there are many candidate solutions and some are better and some are worse than others, but none is clearly best.

be recognized. The implications of the solutions being formulated may similarly take decades to be understood.

A new phenomenon of "known unawareness" has entered our lexicon. In November 2006, Donald Rumsfeld summarized this truth to scattered laughter when he said: "There are known knowns. These are things we know that we know. There are known unknowns. That is to say, there are things that we now know we do not know. But there are also unknown unknowns. These are things we do not know we do not know." (Profita, 2006; https://www.cbsnews.com/news/known-knowns-known-unknowns-and-unknown-unknowns-a-retrospective/). No one is laughing anymore. As a society, we are beginning to realize that despite all we know, the unknown far outweighs what is known. Knowledge is as much to create more questions as it is to provide definitive answers.

Clearly, scientists now know much more about BSE (bovine spongiform encephalopathy or mad cow disease) than when it was first found in cattle in 1986. Even now, decades after the disease's discovery, its origins, its host range, its means of transmission, the nature of the infectious agent, and its relation to its human counterpart new variant Creutzfeldt-Jakob disease remain mostly unknown. We have begun to suspect that there are some risks for which there may be no narrative closure, no ending by which the truth is recovered and the boundaries of the risk established.

Although most of us live and work in nations, our interactions and our risks are increasingly global in nature. The interconnected nature of the global system produces cascading risks at the domestic level. Failing government in Syria produces civil conflict that transfers economic, social, and political pressures into neighboring countries as well as nations around the world. Terrorism threatens the lives of innocent citizens around the world. An oil spill in the Gulf of Mexico reverberates around the world. It becomes increasingly difficult to affix responsibility for problems and their solutions. Who is destroying the ozone, causing global warming, spreading BSE and AIDS? Where did the H5N1 or H1N1 viruses originate and how? Whose responsibility is it to fix these things?

Despite the world's rapid advances in all kinds of sciences, we are increasingly dominated by public perception. Public perception is a palpable force. In some situations, it is an irresistible one. Uncertainties and the risks they give rise to have a social context. Without social and cultural judgments, there are no risks. Nonetheless, these social and cultural judgments are not always grounded in fact. Unfortunately, they are also not always adequately considered in decision-making processes. The public is fond of equating the possibility of an undesirable outcome with the probability of such an outcome. This makes conceivable risks seem very possible, and it fuels our fears of the uncertain. It leads, paradoxically, to audiences that are alternately outraged and indifferent about the risks they face.

Social and cultural views can find and have found their way into public policy. This is in part because many things that were once considered certain and safe, and often vouched for by authorities, turned out to be deadly. The BSE experience in Europe, the SARS (severe acute respiratory syndrome) experience in Asia and elsewhere, the melamine contamination from Chinese products, even ordinary things like dining out or attending a concert provide vivid examples of this phenomenon. Applying knowledge of these experiences to the present and the future devalues the certainties of today. This is what makes conceivable threats seem so possible and what fuels our fears of that which is uncertain. It is also what makes criticism of a decision that masquerades as certain embarrassingly easy.

Responsibility in this more connected world has become less clear. Who has to prove what? What constitutes proof under conditions of uncertainty? What norms of accountability are being used? Who is responsible morally? Who is responsible for paying the costs? These questions plague decision makers nationally and transnationally.

We all live and operate in this uncertain reality. Social values are formed, changed, and re-formed against this backdrop of macro-level uncertainty. There are so many social relationships that it is difficult to know what values the nation, a project area community, or a stakeholder group holds dear at any one point in time. Yet many organizations and individuals cling stubbornly to a deterministic approach to decision making that belies the experience of public and private sectors the world over. Decision making needs a "culture of uncertainty." Risk analysis provides just such a culture.

The future is fundamentally unknowable. There must be recognition of the central importance of demonstrating the collective will to act responsibly and accountably with regard to our efforts to grapple with this fundamental uncertainty and the inevitable shortfalls that will occur despite every best effort to account for this uncertainty. In an uncertain world, we cannot know everything, and we will make mistakes despite our best efforts to the contrary. This is the challenge that invites risk analysis to the fore.

## 2.3    The uncertainty on your desk

The uncertainty that has received the most attention in risk analysis is not the macro-level uncertainty we see from 75,000 feet, nor is it the resulting uncertain environment in which we make decisions. It is the uncertainty that plagues our specific decision contexts. Anyone involved in real problem solving and decision making knows we rarely have all the information we need to make a decision that will yield a certain outcome. For any decision context, we can always make a pile of the things we know and a pile of the things we do not know. For risk analysis, we need to be able to take that pile of things we do not know and sort through it to better understand the nature and causes of the uncertainties we face. It is the nature and cause of the uncertainty that dictates the most appropriate tool to use on it. The first and most important distinction to make in our pile of unknowns is what uncertainty is due to knowledge uncertainty and what is due to natural variability.

## 2.3.1   Knowledge uncertainty or natural variability?

You're headed for Melbourne, Australia, in November and are unsure how to pack because you do not know what the weather is like there at that time of year. For simplicity, let's focus on the daily high temperature. You do not know the mean high temperature for Melbourne in November. This is a parameter, a constant, with a true and factual value. That you do not know this fact makes the situation one of knowledge uncertainty. A true value exists and you do not know it. You are uncertain about a fact.

Suppose you learn from the Bureau of Meteorology, Australia, that this value is 21.9°C (71°F). The knowledge uncertainty has been removed. Now a new problem emerges. Even though you know the average temperature is 21.9°C, you have no way of knowing what the high temperature will be on any given day. In fact, you wisely expect the high temperature to vary from day to day.

---

**DEFINITIONS OF UNCERTAINTY AND VARIABILITY**

*Uncertainty*: Lack or incompleteness of information. Quantitative uncertainty analysis attempts to analyze and describe the degree to which a calculated value may differ from the true value; it sometimes uses probability distributions. Uncertainty depends on the quality, quantity, and relevance of data and on the reliability and relevance of models and assumptions.

*Variability*: Variability refers to true differences in attributes due to heterogeneity or diversity. Variability is usually not reducible by further measurement or study, although it can be better characterized.

**Source: National Research Council (2009)**

---

Using our very loose definition at the start of this chapter, you say you are not sure what the temperature will be on any given day, so that must be uncertainty as well. And in a very general sense it is. However, and this is an important however, this value is uncertain for a very specific, common, and recurring reason; there is natural variability in the universe.

This natural variability is usually separated out from other causes of uncertainty in order to preserve the distinction in its cause for reasons that will soon be apparent. Hence, we'd say you are no longer uncertain about the mean high temperature, but you still do not know the high temperature on any given day because of natural variability. The temperature varies from its mean day to day due to variation in the complex system that produces a high temperature each day. For a more formal distinction of these two concepts, we introduce the terms epistemic and aleatory uncertainty.

Epistemic uncertainty is the uncertainty attributed to a lack of knowledge on the part of the observer. It is reducible in principle, although it may be difficult or expensive to do so. Epistemic uncertainty, what was described in the previous example as knowledge uncertainty, arises from incomplete theory and incomplete understanding of a system, modeling limitations, or limited data. Epistemic uncertainty has also been called internal, functional, subjective, reducible, or model form uncertainty. *Knowledge uncertainty* is another easier to remember and perhaps more descriptive term used to describe this kind of uncertainty. It is used throughout this book when we refer specifically to epistemic uncertainty.

Some generic examples of knowledge uncertainty include lack of experimental data to characterize new materials and processes, poor understanding of the linkages between inputs and outputs in a system, and thinking one value is greater than another but being unsure of that. Other examples include dated, missing, vague, or conflicting information; incorrect methods; faulty models; measurement errors; incorrect assumptions; and the like. Knowledge uncertainty is, quite simply, not knowing a fact. The most common example may be not knowing a parameter or value, like cost or a benefit-cost ratio, that we are interested in for model building or decision-making purposes.

### AN IMPORTANT DISTINCTION

Natural variability cannot be reduced with more or better information.

Knowledge uncertainty can be reduced with more and better information through such means as research, data collection, better modeling and measurement, filling gaps in information and updating out-of-date information, and correcting faulty assumptions.

Aleatory uncertainty is uncertainty that deals with the inherent variability in the physical world. Variability is often attributed to a random process that produces natural variability of a quantity over time and space or among members of a population. It can arise because of natural, unpredictable variation in the performance of the system under study. It is, in principle, irreducible. In other words, the variability cannot be altered by obtaining more information, although one's characterization of that variability might change given additional information. For example, a larger database will provide a more precise estimate of the standard deviation of a temperature, for instance, but it does not reduce variability in the population of daily high temperatures. Aleatory uncertainty is sometimes called variability, irreducible uncertainty, stochastic uncertainty, and random uncertain. The term adopted for usage in this book when we refer specifically to aleatory uncertainty is *natural variability*.

Some generic examples of natural variability include variation in the actual weight of potato chips in an eight-ounce bag, variation in the response of an ecosystem to a change in the physical environment, and variation in hourly traffic counts from day to day. There is also natural variability in any attribute of a population.

*Knowledge uncertainty* and *natural variability* are terms used by the National Research Council (2009). It will be convenient to use the term *uncertainty* to encompass both of these ideas, so that is the convention adopted in this book. However, this is by no means the usual convention, and the reader is advised to always clarify, when possible, and to try to carefully discern, when it is not, what the user of these terms means from the context of their usage.

To complicate matters, reality is often messy. Returning to our Melbourne example, we can see that at the outset we are dealing with both knowledge uncertainty and natural variability. It takes experience for a risk assessor to be able to comfortably label the reasons that a value may be uncertain. It is not always possible and not always important to be able to separate knowledge uncertainty and natural variability. In general, the most important reasons for separating the effects of the two in a risk assessment are to select an appropriate tool for addressing them and to understand that devoting more resources to the risk assessment effort may reduce knowledge uncertainty, but it will not reduce natural variability. The only way to change the natural variability produced by a system is to change the system itself. This will not eliminate natural variability; it will produce a new form of, presumably, more favorable variability in the altered system. Risk assessment can reduce knowledge uncertainty. Risk management measures can alter natural variability.

## 2.3.2   Types of uncertainty

To sort through and understand the nature of the things we do not know, we begin by first differentiating knowledge uncertainty from

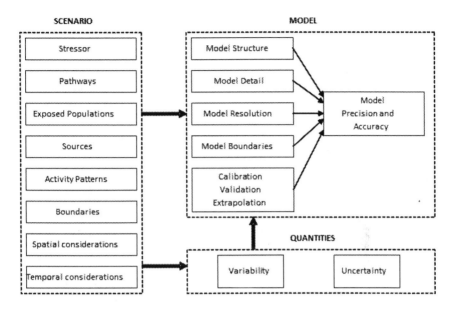

*Figure 2.2* Sorting our knowledge uncertainty into scenarios, models, and input quantities.

natural variability. Natural variability is most often addressed through narrative descriptions of the variability, statistics, and probabilistic methods. Natural variability tends to apply to quantities only. Knowledge uncertainty is a bit more complex and needs additional sorting. The next tier of sorting separates our knowledge uncertainty into scenarios, models, and quantities, as seen in Figure 2.2.

Figure 2.2 provides an example of the types of knowledge uncertainty that might be encountered. It presents an ecological risk example. For now, think of scenarios as the stories we tell about risks. These are the narratives that describe what we believe to be true about the phenomena we study. This is where theory and knowledge of processes are most important. Models are used to give structure to scenarios and to perform calculations based on the quantities provided. Thus, we identify these three broad basic types of knowledge uncertainty you can expect to encounter in risk assessment.

Scenario uncertainty results when the elements of a scenario or their relationships are unknown or incomplete. Gaps in theory and understanding are most likely to occur in the stories we tell about what can go wrong, the consequences of it happening, how it happens, and how likely it is to happen. In the case of an ecosystem scenario, we might misunderstand the stressors that affect a habitat. Not knowing the relevant activity patterns of a locally threatened species could be another source of scenario uncertainty. We may also fail to understand all the relevant pathways in an ecosystem.

Model uncertainty reflects the bias or imprecision associated with compromises made or lack of adequate knowledge in specifying the structure and calibration (parameter estimation) of a model. Model structure typically refers to the set of equations or other functional relationships that comprise the specified scenario for the model. Model detail refers to the inclusion or omission of specific phenomena as well as the simplicity or complexity with which they are represented. Model resolution refers to the temporal or spatial scale at which information can be distinguished, for example, minutes versus hours versus years. Model boundaries describe the fidelity with which the desired scenario is captured by the model. Ideally, the precision and accuracy of the model predictions will be assessed as part of the validation exercise. In other words, how well does our model capture reality?

---

**TYPES OF KNOWLEDGE UNCERTAINTY**

*Scenario uncertainty*: Uncertainty in specifying the risk scenario which is consistent with the scope and purpose of the assessment.

*Model uncertainty*: Uncertainty due to gaps in scientific knowledge which hamper an adequate capture of the correct causal relations between risk factors.

*Parameter/input uncertainty*: Uncertainty involved in the specification of numerical values (be it point values or distributions of values) for the factors which determine the risk.

**Source: WHO (2006)**

---

Quantity or input uncertainty is encountered when the appropriate or true values of quantities are not known (knowledge uncertainty). These quantities are of enough importance to warrant additional discussion.

## 2.3.3   Quantity uncertainty

The most commonly encountered uncertainty is quantity uncertainty. Quantities can be unknown because of knowledge uncertainty or because of natural variability. Morgan and Henrion (1990) offer a very useful taxonomy for those seeking to understand the basic types of quantity uncertainty shown in Figure 2.1. Before considering their taxonomy, we need to make an important distinction. Some quantities have a true or factual value, while others do not. Instead of a true value, they have a best or most appropriate value that reflects some subjective judgment. There may be significant consternation about the best or preferred value for these kinds of quantities, but they have no true value we can discover. The search for a true value is an objective one, while the search for a best value is subjective.

In general, true values are looked up, measured, or estimated by some means. The means by which quantities with true values are estimated vary, and the best choice will depend on the cause of the value's uncertainty. Best or appropriate values are varied systematically (sometimes called parametric variation or sensitivity analysis) to examine the sensitivity of the model and its outputs to different chosen values.

## TRUE VALUES

The population of a city, number of colony forming units per gram of material, percent of channel bottom that is rock, mean strength of materials in a structure, mean daily stream flow, average weight of an adult striped bass, median serving size, specificity of a diagnostic test, closing price of a stock, and contaminant concentration in a specific exposure are all quantities that have a true value.

Risk analysis can require a lot of information. Risk assessment, in particular, can involve a great deal of quantitative information that includes many parameters (numerical constants) and variables. The quantities used in risk assessment are frequently a major source of uncertainty. Having a way to think about these quantities and to talk about their uncertainty is critical to the success of any risk analysis.

Morgan and Henrion's (1990) classification of uncertain quantities includes:

- Empirical quantities
- Defined constants
- Decision variables
- Value parameters
- Index variables
- Model domain parameters
- Outcome criteria

The significance of the objective or subjective nature of the quantity uncertainty, as well as the type of quantity, will become most evident when

*Table 2.1* Uncertain quantity types and examples

| Types of quantities | Selected examples |
| --- | --- |
| Empirical quantities | Stream flow, eggs produced daily, vehicles crossing a bridge, temperature, time to complete a task, prevalence |
| Defined constants | Pi, square feet in an acre, gallons in an acre-foot, speed of light, size of a city |
| Decision variables | Acceptable daily intake, tolerable level of risk, appropriate level of protection, reasonable cost, mitigation goal |
| Value parameters | Value of a statistical life, discount rate, weights assigned in a multicriteria decision analysis, user-day values |
| Index variable | A particular year in a multiyear model, the location of an egg on a pallet, a geographic grid in a spatial model |
| Model domain parameters | Study area, planning horizon, industry segment, climate range |
| Outcome criteria | Mortalities, illness rates, infrastructure failures, fragility curves, costs, probabilities, benefit-cost ratios, risk-risk trade-offs |

one chooses a tool, technique, or methodology to treat the uncertainty appropriately. Look at the examples in Table 2.1, then read the explanations that follow to better understand Morgan and Henrion's taxonomy of quantities. The approach used to resolve uncertainty depends very directly on what is uncertain and why it is uncertain.

### 2.3.3.1   Empirical quantities

Empirical quantities are the most common quantities encountered in a quantitative risk assessment; they have a true value. Empirical quantities are things that can be measured or counted. This includes distances, times, sizes, temperatures, statistics, and any sort of imaginable count. They have exact values that are unknown but measurable in principle, although it may be difficult to do so in practice. A full range of methods from narrative descriptions through probabilistic methods are suitable for addressing uncertainty in these quantities.

### 2.3.3.2   Defined constants

Defined constants have a true value that is fixed by definition. When these values are not known by the analyst, for example, you might not know how many square feet are in an acre or how many gallons of water are in an acre-foot of water, these quantities can end up in the pile of things we do not know. Defined constants provide the perfect opportunity to point out the importance of understanding the nature of your unknowns. When you do not know one of these quantities, you do not use sensitivity analysis or probabilistic methods; instead, you look them up. There are 43,560 square feet in one acre and 325,851 gallons of water in one acre-foot of water.

### 2.3.3.3 Decision variables

This is a quantity which someone must choose or decide. Decision makers exercise direct control over these values; they have no true value. The person deciding this value may or may not be a member of the risk analysis team, depending on the nature of the variable. Policy makers may determine the values of some decision variables to ensure uniformity in decision making. An agency may decide it is unacceptable to increase the lifetime risk of cancer by more than $10^{-6}$, for example. Thus, decision variable values are sometimes set by decision makers external to the risk analysis process.

---

**DECISION RULE UNCERTAINTY**

What is the best endpoint for your purposes? Imprecise or inappropriate operational definitions for desired outcome criteria, for example, "risk," can be a subtle problem.

Concerned about a public health risk? Should you use the number of exposures, infections, illnesses, hospitalizations, or deaths? Which is a better criterion to base a decision on, lifetime mortality risk, annual risk of mortality, risk to children or other subpopulations, or something entirely different?

Concerned about an economic issue? Should you maximize net benefits or minimize costs? Do you want to maximize market share or profits?

There is no right answer to these questions, only better or worse ones. Someone must decide what the decision criterion or rule will be to resolve this uncertainty.

---

In other instances, risk analysis team members may make these decisions. Examples could include determining a tolerable level of risk or design characteristics of risk management options that differentiate one option from another. Decision variables are subjectively determined. Uncertainty about them is most appropriately addressed through parametric variation and sensitivity analysis.

### 2.3.3.4   Value parameters

These values represent aspects of decision makers' preferences and judgments; they have no true value. They are subjective assessments of social values that can describe the values or preferences of stakeholders, the risk manager, or other decision makers. Like decision variables, some of them may be decided by those external to the risk analysis team, while others are decided by team members.

Social values, like the monetary value of a statistical life or society's time preferences for consumption, are likely to be established corporately to ensure uniformity in decision making. Establishing decision-specific values, like assigning relative weights to different decision criteria, may be set by the team. Uncertainty about value parameters is most appropriately addressed through parametric variation and sensitivity analysis.

### 2.3.3.5   Index variables

Index variables identify elements of a model or locations within spatial and temporal domains; they may or may not have a true value. Bacterial counts "24 hours after" yolk membrane breakdown, costs "ten years after" implementing a risk management solution, water quality at a cove, and defining the age and gender of a representative individual are examples of index variables. If a very specific point in time or place in space are desired, there may be a true value. Random or representative choices of index variables do not have true values and are subjectively determined; should we look at future conditions in five years or ten? Uncertainty in index variables is most appropriately addressed through parametric variation and sensitivity analysis.

### 2.3.3.6   Model domain parameters

These values specify and define the scope of the system modeled in a risk assessment. They describe the geographic, temporal, and conceptual boundaries (domain) of a model. They define the resolution of its inputs and outputs; they may or may not have true values. Scale characteristics are chosen by the modeler and most often have no true value in nature. They reflect judgments regarding the model domain and the resolution needed to assess risks adequately. Some risk assessments, however, may be restricted to specific facilities, towns, time frames, and so forth. These may have true values. Uncertainty about domain parameters may also be considered a form of model uncertainty. If the domain is the XYZ processing plant, it is trivially specific and objective. The hinterland affected by economic activity at the Port of Los Angeles is a much more subjective determination. These kinds of quantities are most appropriately addressed through parametric variation and sensitivity analysis.

### 2.3.3.7 Outcome criteria

Outcome criteria, such as illnesses, illnesses prevented, property damage, benefit-cost ratios, and the like, are output variables used to rank or measure the desirability or undesirability of possible decision outcomes. Their values are determined by the input quantities and the models that use them. Uncertainty in these values is evaluated by propagating uncertainty from the input variables to the output variables using one of several different methods. Generating the uncertainty about output criteria is the responsibility of the risk assessor; addressing it in decision making is the responsibility of the risk manager.

## 2.3.4 Sources of uncertainty in empirical quantities

Empirical quantities are the most commonly encountered uncertain quantities with true values that must be measured or estimated. When good measurement data are available, there may be little or no knowledge uncertainty about the true value of a parameter or variable. Even when there is no knowledge uncertainty, we may have natural variability to address in the risk assessment. It is useful to continue the excellent conceptual framework of Morgan and Henrion (1990) to consider the different sources of uncertainty in empirical quantities. Understanding the reasons that you are uncertain about empirical quantities is essential to your ability to choose an effective treatment of that uncertainty in a quantitative risk assessment.

### 2.3.4.1 Random error and statistical variation

Measurements are rarely perfectly exact. Even tiny flaws in observation or reading measuring instruments can cause variations in measurement from one observation to the next. Then there is the statistical variation that results from sample bias. If we take measurements on a sample, we only have an estimate of the true value of a population parameter. Classical statistical techniques provide a wide array of methods and tools for quantifying this kind of uncertainty, including estimators, standard deviations, confidence intervals, hypothesis testing, sampling theory, and probabilistic methods.

### 2.3.4.2 Systematic error and subjective judgment

Systematic errors arise when the measurement instrument, the experiment, or the observer is biased. Imprecise calibration of instruments is one cause of this bias. If the scale is not zeroed or the datum point is off, the solution is better calibration of the instrument or data. If the observer tends to over- or underestimate values, a more objective means of measurement is needed or the observer needs to be recalibrated. The challenge to the risk assessor is to reduce systematic error to a minimum. The best solution is to avoid or correct the bias. When bias can be identified, for example, the scale added 0.1 g to each measurement, it can sometimes be corrected for, that is, by remeasuring or subtracting 0.1 g from each measurement.

---

### IT FEELS LIKE AN EIGHT TO ME

Much data are collected outside a laboratory and under less than ideal conditions. Which box of produce do we open and inspect? Where in the stream does the investigator insert the meter to read dissolved oxygen? How do you estimate how far away a work boat is on the open water? How quickly can you count the deer in a running herd? Subjective judgments are notoriously suspect under uncontrolled conditions.

Just like with faulty instruments, the solution is better calibration. Ideally, before the fact, but calibration is better late than never.

---

The more difficult task concerns the biases that are unknown or merely suspected. Estimating the magnitude of these biases is very difficult and often requires a lot of subjective judgment. Bias in subjective human estimates of unknown quantities is a topic covered extensively in the literature; see, for example, O'Hagan et al. (2006).

### 2.3.4.3   Linguistic imprecision

After all these years on the planet, communication is still humankind's number one challenge. We routinely use the same words to mean different things and different words to mean the same things. This makes communication about complex matters of risk especially challenging. If we say a hazard occurs frequently or a risk is unlikely, what do these words really mean? The problems can be even more pervasive than that. Tasked with measuring the percentage of midday shade on a stream, a group of environmentalists engaged in a lengthy discussion of when midday occurs and how dark must a surface be to be considered shade.

The best and most obvious solution to this kind of ambiguity is to carefully specify all terms and relationships and to clarify all language as it is used. Using quantitative rather than qualitative terms can also help. Fuzzy set theory may be an alternative approach to resolving some of the more unavoidable imprecision of language in a more quantitative fashion.

### 2.3.4.4 Natural variability

Many quantities vary over time, space, or from one individual or object in a population to another. This variability is inherent in the system that produces the population of things we measure. Frequency distributions based on samples or probability distributions for populations, if available, can be used to estimate the values of interest. Other probabilistic methods may also be used.

### 2.3.4.5 Randomness and unpredictability

Inherent randomness is sometimes singled out as a form of uncertainty different from all others, in part because it is irreducible in principle. The indeterminacy of Heisenberg's uncertainty principle is one example of inherent randomness. However, a valid argument could be made that this is just another instance of knowledge uncertainty because we simply have been unable to resolve this puzzle at the present time.

This cause of uncertainty identifies those uncertainties that are not predictable in practice at the current time. Examples include such things as when the next flood will occur on a stream or where the next food-borne outbreak will occur in the United States. Such events can be treated as a legitimately random process. The danger here is the personalist view of randomness that could emerge, where randomness is a function of the risk assessor's knowledge. Phenomena that appear random to one assessor may be the result of a process well known by a subject-matter expert. Strong interdisciplinary risk assessment teams combined with peer involvement and peer review processes provide a reasonable hedge against this sort of problem arising. Uncertainty about such quantities can be addressed by a full range of methods, from narrative descriptions through probabilistic methods.

### 2.3.4.6 Disagreement

Organizations and experts do not always see eye to eye on matters of uncertainty. Different technical interpretations of the same data can give rise to disagreements, as can widely disparate views of the problem. This is not to mention the real possibility of conscious or unconscious motivational bias.

Disagreements can sometimes be resolved through negotiation and other issue resolution techniques. Allowing the disagreements to coexist is also an option. Sensitivity analysis would consider the results of the analysis using each different perspective. A common approach for some disagreements is to combine the judgments using subjective weights.

### 2.3.4.7  *Approximation*

There may be instances when it is useful to approximate values of one quantity with another quantity. This is sometimes done with microbial dose-response curves where values for one species are used to approximate values for another species. Uncertainty due to approximation is also similar to what we called model uncertainty, earlier in this chapter. The fact that the model is a simplified version of reality ensures that uncertainty will remain about the outcome criteria. We are only able to approximate the function of complex systems because of scenario, model, and quantity uncertainty. Methods for dealing with this source of uncertainty will depend on the specific limitations of the approximation.

## 2.4  *Being intentional about uncertainty*

Risk analysis is decision making under uncertainty. It requires risk assessors, risk managers, and risk communicators to become intentional about uncertainty. Here are 10 actions to take to become intentional about uncertainty in decision making:

1. Recognize that uncertainty exists and is relevant in your decision problem.
2. Identify the specific things that are uncertain and the sources of that uncertainty.
3. Identify the instrumental uncertainties among the uncertainty. These are the uncertainties that have the potential to affect the decision or decision outcomes.
4. Acknowledge the relevant uncertainty and make risk managers, other decision makers, and stakeholders aware of instrumental uncertainties.
5. Choose appropriate tools and techniques to address each source of instrumental uncertainty.
6. Complete the assessment and other analyses incorporating these tools and techniques.
7. Understand the results of the uncertainty analysis.
8. Identify any options for further reducing the remaining instrumental uncertainty.
9. Convey the results and the significance of the instrumental uncertainty for decision making and decision outcomes, as well as any options for reducing the residual uncertainty, to decision makers in a manner that enables them to use this information in decision making.
10. Proclaim the uncertainty and its potential impacts on decision outcomes to all appropriate stakeholders.

The process begins by recognizing uncertainty when it exists and it almost always exists. It is not unusual for experienced professionals to underestimate the things they do not know or to overestimate the quality of their evidence. Experts are often confident, not so much because of what they actually know as what they believe to be true. Biases, mindsets, and beliefs can prevent some people from recognizing that uncertainty exists. Experts are often correct in their intuitive judgments and this strongly reinforces those biases. Thus, the starting point for all risk work is to begin by recognizing the existence of uncertainty. This may, at times, require analysts to challenge one another. To challenge false beliefs in certainty, ask: "What is your evidence for your beliefs about this problem?" When experts can produce evidence, it is reassuring. When they cannot, it can be enlightening.

### ROCK IN THE CHANNEL

During one proof-of-concept, risk-based estimate of costs in the early 1990s, a design engineer was asked to estimate the percentage of rock in a channel bottom with an estimated interval. He declined to do so and, when pressed, he refused. His justification was that he had much more and much better data than he normally has. He was offended by the notion that he might not know how much rock was actually in the channel bottom. His point estimate proved to be off by a significant amount. He has become a supporter of interval estimates.

Once the existence of uncertainty is recognized, it is necessary to specifically identify what is known with certainty and what is not. The analyst's job is to identify those uncertain things that are most important to decision making. These would be scenarios, theories and knowledge, models or quantities that if not certain could affect decision making or decision outcomes. It is not unusual to find many potential sources of uncertainty. Some of these will be more important than others and risk assessors and other analysts need to be able to identify uncertainties that are instrumental from those that are not. Risk managers do not need to be concerned with every potential uncertainty. In some instances, instrumental uncertainties may not be identified until after the assessment is completed.

There are going to be people who need to know about the uncertainty perhaps even before you begin to address it. Consider a large public works project, where design engineers are uncertain about the existence of seismic zones in the project footprint. This could affect the work of cost estimators and others who need to know this. Acknowledging the known uncertainties early in the assessment process is an important first step in risk communication. Partners in the decision-making process are certainly going to need to know the limitations of the available data.

Matching an appropriate tool and technique to the uncertainty is an important analytical step. Some uncertainty can be addressed in a qualitative risk assessment. Other uncertainty may require a probabilistic risk assessment. Between and beyond these approaches lie many tools and techniques.

Characterizing the risks and the uncertainty that is associated with them for a decision problem requires analysts to pull together the many and disparate approaches for addressing uncertainty that may have been used and to complete the analyses. It is important for the analysts to spend sufficient time with the results of their analyses to understand them and the uncertainty that attends them well enough to explain its implications for decision making and decision outcomes to risk managers and other decision makers.

In best practice, analysts will be able to distinguish the effects of knowledge uncertainty from the effects of natural variability. This will enable the analyst to identify potential options for further reducing the uncertainty in the risk assessment and other analyses. One of the greatest challenges, and an area of risk analysis that has not yet received sufficient attention, is to convey the results, the significance of the uncertainty, and any options for reducing uncertainty to decision makers. This is the subject of Chapter 7 on decision making under uncertainty.

It is the risk assessor's responsibility to identify and address the instrumental uncertainty in their decision problems. Some of the simpler tools available include narrative descriptions of the uncertainty, clarification of ambiguous language, negotiation for differences of opinion, and uncertainty or confidence ratings for these analyses. When the relevant uncertainty could lead to dramatically different futures and a few key drivers of this uncertainty can be identified, scenario planning is a useful technique. In more quantitative analyses, assessors can use parametric variation, bound uncertain values, and use sensitivity analysis or other quantitative risk assessment methods, all of which can include both deterministic and probabilistic analysis.

It is the decision maker's responsibility as risk manager to address instrumental uncertainty in decision making. In order to do that, risk assessors must make sure decision makers, in their risk management responsibility, understand the potential for instrumental uncertainty to affect decision making or the potential outcomes of any specific decision. Chapter 7 provides a practical approach for risk managers to follow in addressing instrumental uncertainty in decision making. It also includes a discussion of criteria that have been developed for choosing from among alternative risk management measures under uncertainty. They include:

- Maximax criterion—choosing the option with the best upside payoff.
- Maximin criterion—choosing the option with the best downside payoff.
- Laplace criterion—choosing the option based on expected value payoff.
- Hurwicz criterion—choosing an option based on a composite score derived from preference weights assigned to selected values (e.g., the maximum and minimum).
- Regret (minimax) criterion—choosing the option that minimizes the maximum regret associated with each option.

Once a decision is made, the potential impacts of uncertainty on the decision's outcomes must be vigorously proclaimed to all stakeholders with a legitimate interest in knowing how they may be affected by the decision and the uncertainty that attends it. Making this effort to be honest brokers of information, saying what we do and do not know, and stating the significance of the latter for decision making distinguishes risk analysis from other decision-support frameworks and tools. As Figure 2.3 shows, the uncertainty encountered in an assessment of a risk can be found in either its probability or consequence. It can be due to knowledge uncertainty or natural variability. It is the risk assessors' responsibility to address significant relevant uncertainties in their assessments. Risk managers are expected to address instrumental uncertainty in their decision making.

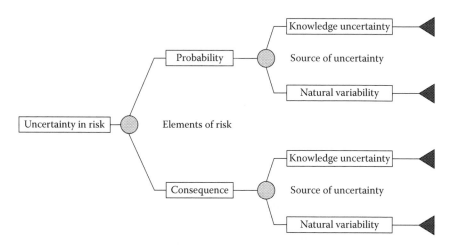

*Figure 2.3* Source elements of uncertainty in risk analysis.

## 2.5 Summary and look forward

Uncertainty is the reason for risk analysis. Risk analysis is, in a sense, the confluence of social values and science. Uncertainty at the macro-level affects values through a constantly and rapidly changing social environment. Uncertainty at the micro-level occurs in the specific details of the problems decision makers face, at the level of our scientific knowledge. The two levels of uncertainty can pose markedly different challenges to risk analysts.

Separating what we know from what we do not know is a primary responsibility of the risk assessor. In the "pile of things" we do not know about a given decision problem are things that reflect our knowledge uncertainty and things that are naturally variable. It is important to know the difference between the two. Knowledge uncertainty is, in principle, reducible, while natural variability is not. This can be important to how risks are assessed, managed, and communicated.

A major purpose of risk analysis is to push risk assessors and risk managers to be intentional in how they address uncertainty in assessment and decision making. There are helpful taxonomies to aid our thinking about how to identify uncertainties and their causes. These are important to know because different kinds and causes of uncertainty have different sets of appropriate treatments. It is the risk assessor's job to address knowledge uncertainty and natural variability in risk assessment inputs. It is the risk manager's job to address them in risk assessment outputs.

The next three chapters will carefully unpack and explain the basic activities that comprise the three components of the risk analysis model presented in Chapter 1. We begin with the risk management process, which is the cornerstone of the risk analysis process. Although there are many well-developed risk management models already in use, the approach taken here is not to put any one of these before the others so much as to find the common ground in all of them to aid your understanding and practice of the risk management process.

## References

Morgan, M. G., and M. Henrion. 1990. *Uncertainty: A guide to dealing with uncertainty in quantitative risk and policy analysis.* Cambridge, UK: Cambridge University Press.

National Research Council. 2009. *Committee on improving risk analysis approaches used by the U.S. EPA. Advancing risk assessment 2009.* Washington, DC: National Academies Press.

O'Hagan, A., C. E. Buck, A. Daneshkhah, J. R. Eiser, P. H. Garthwaite, D. J. Jenkinson, J. E. Oakley, and T. Rakow. 2006. *Uncertain judgments: Eliciting experts" probabilities.* West Sussex, UK: John Wiley & Sons.

Profita, H. 2006. Known knowns, known unknowns and unknown unknowns: A retrospective. CBS News. https://www.cbsnews.com/news/known-knowns-known-unknowns-and-unknown-unknowns-a-retrospective/ (accessed October 31, 2018).

Tainter, J. A. 1996. *Getting down to earth: Practical applications of ecological economics.* Washington, DC: Island Press.

World Economic Forum. 2018. *The Global Risks Report 2018*, 13th edition. Geneva. ISBN: 978-1-944835-15-6.

World Health Organization. International Programme on Chemical Safety. 2006. *Part 1: Guidance document on characterizing and communicating uncertainty in exposure assessment.* Geneva: World Health Organization. https://www.who.int/ipcs/methods/harmonization/areas/uncertainty%20.pdf (accessed January 8, 2019).

# *chapter three*

# *Risk management*

## *3.1 Introduction*

In the past, many organizations have managed risks by prescribing standards, policy, procedures, regulations, and other guidance, the rationale being that if you follow the "rules," then whatever results must be okay. That is not risk management. Risk management, done well, is intentional about its process, addresses uncertainty in decision making, and focuses on outcomes. Risk management is maturing. There are now thousands of people who identify themselves as risk managers when only a few decades ago few outside of the insurance industry used this title.

There is no shortage of risk management models. As with every other aspect of risk analysis, many disciplines and organizations have spawned their own particular view of how to do risk management. Describing the risk management process in a generic fashion is, therefore, a daunting challenge. It is impossible to define risk management in a way that will satisfy many, much less all, people. The Society for Risk Analysis defines it benignly as "Activities to handle risk such as prevention, mitigation, adaptation or sharing." It is not a lack of definitions that makes defining the term difficult so much as it is the proliferation of definitions in use by organizations and found in the literature. The U.S. Environmental Protection Agency's *Thesaurus of Terms Used in Microbial Risk Assessment*, for example, identifies 12 different definitions for risk management (EPA, 2010).

It goes without saying that most organizations are quite fond of the nuances or parsimony of their own definitions and are not inclined to surrender it for another. No one seems to be clamoring for a universal definition, so do not look for one here. In place of a formal definition, the risk management component is described in some detail. That description will not be any more universally applicable than a definition would be, but we must begin somewhere, so we begin by identifying those risk management activities that are common to many definitions, models, and practice.

**A SAMPLING OF RISK MANAGEMENT DEFINITIONS**

The culture, processes, and structures that are directed toward the effective management of potential opportunities and adverse effects. (Australia/New Zealand Risk Standard)

The sum of measures instituted by people or organizations in order to reduce, control, and regulate risks. (German Advisory Council on Global Change)

Decision-making process involving considerations of political, social, economic, and technical factors with relevant risk assessment information relating to a hazard so as to develop, analyze, and compare regulatory and nonregulatory options and to select and implement appropriate regulatory response to that hazard. Risk Management involves three elements: risk evaluation; emission and exposure control; risk monitoring. (IPCS)

Coordinated activities to direct and control an organization with regard to risk. (ISO/IEC Risk Management Vocabulary)

All the processes involved in identifying, assessing and judging risks, assigning ownership, taking actions to mitigate or anticipate them, and monitoring and reviewing progress. Good risk management helps reduce hazard and builds confidence to innovate. (UK Government Handling Risk Report)

The process of analyzing, selecting, implementing, and evaluating actions to reduce risk. (US Presidential/Congressional Commission)

The process of evaluating alternative regulatory actions and selecting among them. (U.S. National Research Council "Red Book")

I am going to call a new initiative undertaken by an organization that practices risk analysis, a risk management activity. There are five basic parts to a risk management activity, all connected by continuing risk communication. The five parts are:

1. Identifying risk
2. Estimating risk
3. Evaluating risk
4. Controlling risk
5. Monitoring risk

A generic model is shown in Figure 3.1. It shows the five parts in a continuous loop in order to capture the iterative nature of risk

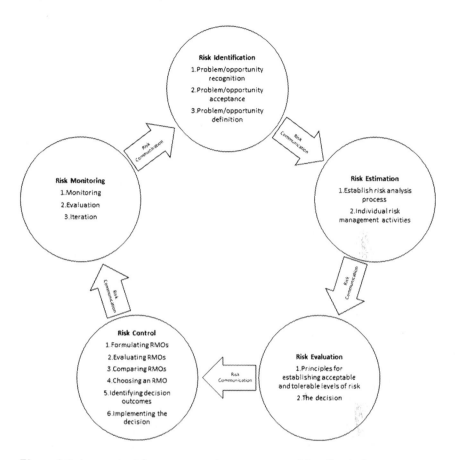

**Risk Identification**

1. Problem/opportunity recognition
2. Problem/opportunity acceptance
3. Problem/opportunity definition

**Risk Estimation**

1. Establish risk analysis process
2. Individual risk management activities

**Risk Evaluation**

1. Principles for establishing acceptable and tolerable levels of risk
2. The decision

**Risk Control**

1. Formulating RMOs
2. Evaluating RMOs
3. Comparing RMOs
4. Choosing an RMO
5. Identifying decision outcomes
6. Implementing the decision

**Risk Monitoring**

1. Monitoring
2. Evaluation
3. Iteration

*Figure 3.1* A generic risk management process comprising five tasks.

management. Risk management is making effective and practical decisions under conditions of uncertainty. As long as there is any uncertainty, a risk management decision is conditional, that is, based on what was known and not known at the time of the decision. As the uncertainty is reduced in the future or as the outcomes of the management decision become known, it may be prudent to revise the decision, hence, the ongoing nature of risk management. Every decision is based on what we know now and is subject to further revision in the future; in that sense, no decision is necessarily final as long as instrumental uncertainty remains. Expanding on and explaining the elements of the risk management model of Figure 3.1 is the primary work of this chapter.

You will find this to be a wide-ranging chapter, as befits the risk manager's job. I have distilled the most consistent elements of a great many risk management models (see e.g., Presidential/Congressional

Commission, 1997; FAO, 2003; FDA, 2003a; ISO, 2009), as well as my own experience, to the five broad parts of a risk management activity, which are described here in some detail. To round out the discussion, a few specific risk management models are offered at the end of the chapter to illustrate how different organizations approach the risk management task, which is basically to make effective decisions about whether and how to manage risks with less than all the information desired.

## 3.2   *Identifying risks*

Something happens to start a risk management activity. That something is usually a problem that needs attention or an opportunity* that can be pursued. In Chapter 1, a risk identification process consisting of the following steps was identified:

- Identify the trigger event.
- Identify the hazard or opportunity for uncertain gain.
- Identify the specific harm or harms that could result from the hazard or opportunity for uncertain gain.
- Specify the sequence of events that is necessary for the hazard or opportunity for uncertain gain to result in the identified harm(s).
- Identify the most significant uncertainties in the preceding steps.

In this expanded discussion it will be convenient to think of risks a little differently, as problems and opportunities.

Einstein is reported to have said, "If I had one hour to save the world, I would spend 55 minutes defining the problem." This is the stake that good risk analysis drives into the ground at its outset that helps distinguish it from other decision-making paradigms. The purpose of risk analysis is to find the right problem and to solve it. Identifying the problem (see Figure 3.2) provides a focal point for all of the risk manager's subsequent decision-making efforts.

What often happens in organizations is that as soon as a problem arises, we are so eager to solve it that we spend very little time understanding, refining, and communicating our understanding of it. As a consequence, organizations often treat the symptoms of problems rather than their causes. Worse, we often do not even know when we are unclear about a problem, and frequently the result is that we solve the "wrong" problem correctly.

---

* To avoid the awkward redundancy of saying problem/opportunity throughout this section, let it be understood that problem will stand for both kinds of risky situations.

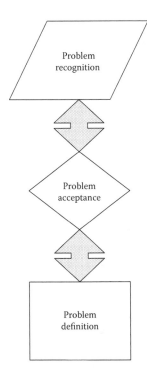

*Figure 3.2* Problem identification steps.

**EXAMPLES OF TRIGGERS FOR RISK MANAGEMENT ACTIVITIES**

*Crisis*: Real or perceived, media, public outcry, adverse comments, changing public values or awareness, decreased consumer confidence, other.

*Science and technology*: New knowledge or technology, emerging health problem, improved detection, surveillance, or method.

*Emerging or "on the horizon"*: Planned search, forecasting, scan risk landscape, natural and anthropogenic disasters and events, imports.

*Strategic plan*: Strategic planning, social needs, opportunities, can be beyond the horizon, historical precedents.

These examples of the kinds of events and inputs that can trigger a risk management activity are from the Food and Drug Administration (FDA) *Center for Food Safety and Applied Nutrition Risk Management Framework* (FDA, 2003a).

Problem identification, the risk manager's first major responsibility, is defined here as a three-part process (see Figure 3.2).

- Problem recognition
- Problem acceptance
- Problem definition

## 3.2.1   Problem recognition

Problem recognition is the simple act of recognizing that a problem exists and gaining an initial understanding of the problem. This happens in one of two broad ways. Reactive or passive problem recognition is when a problem finds you. These are problems triggered by outside influences. Stakeholders bring you a problem or an event occurs that results in a problem you cannot ignore. Alternatively, there is proactive or intentional problem finding, in which management looks actively and often strategically for the most important problem(s) to solve.

Despite the seemingly obvious nature of this task, it is surprising how frequently organizations fail to recognize a problem. This is all the truer in a risk analysis context because risky problems often lurk unseen over the horizon or around the corner. They are frequently hidden from view, obscured by uncertainty and higher priorities, and occluded by smoke from the organizational brushfires that need constant tamping out. Anyone can recognize the problem that forces its way through your door and onto your desk at 4 p.m. on a Friday afternoon. It takes a risk manager to see the problems just over the horizon or just around the corner.

Recognizing the existence of opportunities for potential gain or betterment parallels the process of problem recognition. Fewer opportunities seem to break down the risk manager's door than do problems, however, and the search for opportunities is usually more active.

## 3.2.2   Problem acceptance

Once a problem makes your radar screen, the question becomes, "Will you own it and do something about it?" The second step in problem identification, therefore, is problem acceptance. This requires risk managers to articulate the problem they have found in enough detail to determine if it is a problem they are willing and able to address. Addressing a problem means allocating resources to its solution.

Risk managers must identify the resources required to address the problem in a timely manner. Then they must evaluate the adequacy of their available resources in the context of their program authorities, organizational mission, and vision. This obviously implies consideration of competing uses for the organization's resources. We cannot solve every problem.

Problem acceptance is a priority-setting step. It is deciding to act. Accepting a problem as one to be solved or an opportunity as one to be pursued is a significant organizational commitment. Our understanding of the problem is revised and refined beyond the initial recognition in this step. Risk managers must identify and commit to the time frame and resources required to address each problem they accept.

Choosing from a number of potential opportunities and deciding which are worth pursuing is a common challenge in business decision making. Articulating and accepting the opportunities to be pursued parallels the problem acceptance step.

### 3.2.3 Problem definition

The third step is problem definition. This is when the problem is fully articulated for the first time and linked to possible solutions. Opportunities are likewise articulated and linked to potential strategies that could realize the gains. Information needs begin to become clear and a risk management activity is initiated. This step encompasses a focused and intentional effort to provide a commonly understood description of the problem. It includes stakeholder input when appropriate.

If you cannot clearly and concisely finish the sentence, "The problem is …," then nothing that follows will be clear either. A written "problems and opportunities statement" is the desired output of this problem identification process. Your problems and opportunities statement provides the rationale or reason for your risk management activity. It should be considered a conditional statement that will change as you begin to gather information, reduce the initial uncertainty, and better understand the problem(s) and stakeholders' concerns. So, date that piece of paper. Risk analysis is an iterative process and you can expect to revise and refine your problems and opportunities statement several times before you are done.

---

**SAMPLE PROBLEMS AND OPPORTUNITIES STATEMENT**

P1: Increasing resistance of *Campylobacter* in chicken to fluoroquinolones due to subtherapeutic use of antibiotic drugs in food producing animals.

P2: Declining efficacy in the use of fluoroquinolones for the treatment of fluoroquinolone-resistant campylobacteriosis in humans.

O1: Reduce incidence of all campylobacteriosis in humans due to consumption of chicken.

The stakeholders in any problem context will vary. For some problems, the stakeholders may comprise the general public and many special interests. In other problem settings the stakeholders may be wholly contained within the risk managing organization. Stakeholders, however defined, should be involved in the problem identification process. The appropriate level of involvement will vary with the decision problem and its context. Some problems will be identified for you by stakeholders; at other times they will have to be made aware of the existence of a problem.

Vet your problems and opportunities statement with your stakeholders. Publish it appropriately. Make it public if your stakeholders include members of the public. Show them your best thinking and ask, "Did we get the problem(s) right? What is missing? What is here that should not be? Do you have information about these problems and opportunities that would be helpful to share?" Stakeholders can be an effective ally in reducing uncertainty.

The output of this activity is a revised problems and opportunities statement. Keep that statement up to date. Let people know how it changes and why it changes as it changes.

### 3.2.4   From problems and opportunities to risks

Given a problems and opportunities statement, it is straightforward to identify the risks to be addressed in a decision. Very often, the statement itself will suffice as a summary identification of risks. However, for clarity, it would be wise to expand each problem and opportunity using the risk identification steps presented at the outset of this section, described in detail in Section 1.2.

## 3.3   Risk estimation

Estimating risks is the assessor's job. It cannot be done without direction and guidance from the risk manager. Risk managers have an important, but limited, role in the science-based risk assessment process. The risk manager's positive decision-making role is found in the risk estimation activities (see Figure 3.3) that help describe the world as it actually is. That role includes establishing the organization's risk analysis process and managing individual risk management activities.

There are two groups of activities in the risk estimation part of risk management, as seen in Figure 3.3. The first, developing a risk analysis process, consists of one-time or periodic activities required to establish and maintain the risk analysis process. The other, individual risk management activities, consists of duties that recur in every risk management activity. These activities are addressed below at the level of detail shown in the figure.

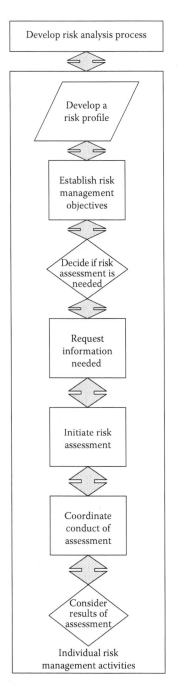

*Figure 3.3* Risk estimation steps.

Recommendation 1 from the U.S. National Research Council (NRC) publication *Risk Assessment in the Federal Government: Managing the Process,* also known as the "Red Book," has been often misunderstood to mean that the assessment and management tasks must be functionally separated and should not interact. The actual recommendation follows.

> Regulatory agencies should take steps to establish and maintain a clear conceptual distinction between assessment of risks and the consideration of risk management alternatives; that is, the scientific findings and policy judgments embodied in risk assessments should be explicitly distinguished from the political, economic, and technical considerations that influence the design and choice of regulatory strategies
>
> **Source: NRC (1983)**

That is a far cry from the severe separation that has been practiced at times.

### 3.3.1   Establish a risk analysis process

If the plethora of definitions for the basic terminology of risk analysis teaches us nothing else, it teaches us this: there is no one best way to do risk analysis. The most commonsense rule seems to be to use what works best for you. Think of risk analysis as a process that is firm in its principles but flexible in the details of how they are pursued.

The risk manager's job, with respect to establishing a risk analysis process, is basically to say, "This is how we do risk analysis here." This process establishes the risk management model the organization will use so that there is an agreed-upon framework for addressing risk problems and opportunities. It establishes the roles and responsibilities of everyone involved in the risk analysis process.

A significant piece of any risk analysis process is the risk assessment policy, which addresses the manner in which the many subjective judgments and choices that arise in the course of a risk assessment will be resolved to protect the integrity of the science and the decision-making process. Some predictable issues that will arise include how to deal with uncertainty and what assumptions to use when the available data are inconsistent. These are sometimes called "science policy" issues. It is wise to devise a means of identifying and resolving these kinds of problems before they are encountered in practice.

Establishing a risk assessment policy is the risk manager's responsibility. It needs to be a collaborative process for any organization that is engaged in making public policy or in the stewardship of public resources like public health, public safety, natural resources, or the environment. This collaboration should include risk managers, risk assessors, and risk communicators. It should provide appropriate opportunities for input and feedback from relevant stakeholders. The risk assessment policy should be documented and made publicly available to ensure consistency, clarity, and transparency. For most organizations outside the public sector, establishing a risk assessment policy is an internal affair.

## SCIENCE POLICY

Risk assessors might be faced with several scientifically plausible approaches (for example, choosing the most reliable dose-response model for extrapolation beyond the range of observable effects) with no definitive basis for distinguishing among them. The [Red Book] committee pointed out that selection of a particular approach under such circumstances involves what it called a science-policy choice. Science-policy choices are distinct from the policy choices associated with ultimate decision making... The science-policy choices that regulatory agencies make in carrying out risk assessments have considerable influence on the results

**Source: NRC (1983)**

When the science is unclear, what assumptions are to be made and by whom? A good risk assessment policy addresses these questions and all questions of "so-called" default assumptions.

One of the hallmarks of best-practice risk analysis is insulating the science from the policy. In the early days of risk analysis, many thought the risk management and risk assessment tasks must be totally separated from one another. This is not true. It is best when these functions are separate and handled by different people with the appropriate skill sets required by their jobs. However, it is absolutely essential that managers and assessors communicate, cooperate, and even, at times, collaborate throughout the risk analysis process.

---

**A SCALABLE PROCESS**

A good risk management process is perfectly scalable. You can use it when you have 30 minutes and no budget as easily as you can over years with millions of dollars.

Its greatest value is that it provides a systematic, science-based approach to solving problems and managing risks.

---

Risk managers begin and end the risk assessment process. They may collaborate with risk assessors in identifying a problem, in formulating risk management options, or on other tasks throughout the risk management activity. They will cooperate in the conduct of the risk assessment and must communicate continuously throughout the iterative risk analysis process.

The output of this task is a well-defined risk analysis process that will guide the organization. That process should include a specific risk management model and a risk assessment policy. Both of these should be carefully documented and publicized to all those with a legitimate interest in the organization's risk analysis process.

## 3.3.2   Individual risk management activities

Risk managers have several specific preliminary risk management responsibilities to complete before, during, and after the risk assessment. Identifying the right problem to solve is only the starting point. Additional responsibilities include:

1. Develop a risk profile
2. Establish risk management objectives
3. Decide if a risk assessment is needed
4. Request needed information
5. Initiate the risk assessment
6. Coordinate the conduct of the assessment
7. Consider the results of the assessment

Each of these activities is considered in turn in the following sections.

### 3.3.2.1 Develop a risk profile

Risk profile is a term with two distinctly different meanings. In its current context, it is an initial data-gathering effort. In an enterprise risk management (ERM) context, a risk profile is something between a description of a set of risks of concern to an organization (and, thus, not markedly different from this current context) and a high-level assessment of the types of risks an organization faces. Be aware, this is a potentially confusing term. The ERM context of the term is revisited at length in Chapter 6.

Once the problems have been articulated in a problems and opportunities statement, it is time to quickly find out what is and is not known about the decision problem. A risk profile presents an analysis of the types of risks an organization, asset, project, or individual faces based on available information. In the current context, a risk profile frames problems and opportunities in their risk context and provides as much information as possible to guide subsequent risk assessment, risk management, and risk communication activities. It also provides the first formal identification of the uncertainty in your decision problem.

**INFORMATION YOU MIGHT FIND IN A RISK PROFILE**
- Latest statement of the problem
- Description of the hazard or opportunity involved
- How assets are exposed to the hazard
- Frequency, distribution, and levels of occurrence of the hazard
- Identification of possible risks from the available scientific literature
- Nature of values at risk (human health, economic, cultural, etc.)
- Distribution of the risk and benefits from the risky activity
- High level or preliminary assessment or prioritization of the risks
- Characteristics of available risk management options
- Current risk management practices relevant to the issue
- Public perceptions of the potential risks
- Information about possible risk management (control) measures
- Preliminary identification of important scientific data gaps that may prevent or limit a risk assessment
- International implications of risk management
- Risk management objectives
- Decision to pursue a risk assessment
- Questions to be answered by risk assessment

The risk profile is the risk manager's responsibility. Managers need not do it alone or at all, for that matter, but they need to see that it is done. Profiling a risk will almost surely mean consulting and collaborating with risk assessors, and it may involve stakeholders. The preliminary risk identification is fleshed out and expanded upon in the profile. Think of this as the point at which the risk management activity team provides a situation report based on available evidence and information that more carefully develops our understanding of what can go wrong, how it can happen, the consequences of it happening, and how likely it is to happen. The profile presents the current state of knowledge related to the risks identified in a concise form at the outset of the risk management activity. The profile will also include consideration of potential risk management options identified to date.

The profile step is important for several reasons beyond the fact that it identifies data gaps by separating what we initially know about a problem or opportunity from what we do not know. It develops the risk analysis team's knowledge and understanding of the problem and may evolve the risk identification further. It also provides the basis for some very important preliminary risk management tasks including:

- Identifying risk management objectives
- Deciding whether or not to initiate a risk assessment
- Identifying the questions to be answered by risk assessment

One of the most important functions of the risk profile is to reduce and better define the uncertainty relevant to the decision problem. When a risk is initially identified, it is likely that the uncertainty is going to be great. As the first formal information-gathering step in the process, the risk profile is often effective in reducing uncertainty and identifying the greatest remaining data gaps. A risk profile sometimes provides enough information to make a risk management decision.

The term *risk profile* is used extensively by the food safety risk analysis community, for one example. It may be an unfamiliar term to other communities of practice. However, the initial data-gathering step is or should be universal in any risk management activity. Finding out what is already known or readily knowable about the identified risks precedes the risk assessment. In fact, it is an essential step in deciding whether a risk assessment is even needed or in some instances whether it is doable.

The output of this step is a documented risk profile that includes the initial sorting and assessing of the things that are not known about the identified problems and opportunities. Documentation may be in a brief report, an organized sheaf of papers, an electronic folder of information sources and memoranda, or an oral narrative. A formal document is not always required.

### 3.3.2.2 Establish risk management objectives

Objectives say what we desire to see happen and when. They define what success looks like. An objective is a clear statement of a desired outcome of the risk management activity. It is easy to confuse objectives with strategies, which describe how we intend to achieve the objectives. It is the risk manager's job to write the risk management objectives. They should be specific and conceptually measurable.

**SAMPLE OBJECTIVE WORDS**

Eliminate, reduce, minimize/maximize, enhance, harmonize, identify, define, describe, increase/decrease, raise/lower, strengthen/ weaken, avoid, adapt, blend, reconcile, coordinate, affirm, diminish, weaken, promote, raise, complement, strengthen.

Once the risk has been profiled and the decision context is better understood, risk managers need to determine their broad risk management objectives. The problems and opportunities statement describes why a risk management activity has been initiated. The objectives state in broad and general terms what the risk managers intend to do about the problems and opportunities they face. These objectives should reflect the most important social (or organizational) values in the decision process.

**A GOOD OBJECTIVE IS**

*Specific*: It is clear and free from ambiguity
*Flexible*: It can be adapted to new or changing requirements
*Measurable*: Its achievement can be documented by some objective
   means
*Attainable*: It can be reached at the end of a course of action
*Congruent*: It is in harmony with other objectives
*Acceptable*: It is welcome or pleasing to key stakeholders

Objectives do not identify specific risk management options, they are not solutions to the problem(s) identified. They identify the intended purposes of the risk management activity. An objective is a clear statement of a desired end that risk management options are intended to accomplish.

Where do these objectives come from? Values! They reflect what is important to people. You can find values in what concerns the public, the experts, and our institutions (law, regulations, guidance, policy, organizational missions).

**A GOOD OBJECTIVE IS NOT A**

*Management option*: It does not prescribe a specific course of action
*Government goal*: It is not a political or governmental objective
*Risk assessment task*: Developing a dose-response curve is not an objective
*Resource constraint*: It does not address time, money, or expertise
*Absolute target*: It does not specify a particular level of achievement

Consider a risk management objective related to a health risk. The objective may be to reduce or eliminate the health risk. An objective does not say how that can or should be done, only that it is an objective to do so. Objectives related to economic values might include increasing jobs, income, and profits or minimizing costs. Objectives related to other public values might include things like protecting children or the environment.

Objectives reflect the most important social (or organizational) values in the decision-making process. They identify the things risk managers are trying to do. Sometimes, there are important things we are trying not to do. These things we will call constraints. Examples of constraints include not creating new risks, avoiding the loss of jobs or income, and avoiding negative impacts on endangered and threatened species. Constraints, as used here, should not be confused with resource or schedule limitations.

A formal and written objectives and constraints statement is the desired output of this task. Consider it conditional and subject to change as uncertainty is reduced and you iterate your way through the risk management activity.

This is one of the critical ways in which social values are appropriately reflected in the risk analysis process. Stakeholder input is essential for identifying good objectives and constraints. Like the problems and opportunities statement, this statement should be published and vetted as appropriate to the decision problem's context. Seek input to the formation of these objectives and ask for feedback on your statement. Not every risk management activity is going to require the same kind of review process. Private organizations making internal decisions may require no public involvement, while some government organizations may require extensive public involvement.

**SAMPLE OBJECTIVES AND CONSTRAINTS STATEMENT**

O1: Reduce *Campylobacter* antimicrobial resistance to fluoroquinolones.

O2: Reduce the number of cases of human illness due to resistant *Campylobacter* in chicken.

O3: Support the economic viability of chicken production.

O4: Improve animal welfare in chicken production.

C1: Do not increase the number of non-fluoroquinolone resistant cases of Campylobacteriosis.

The success of a risk management activity is defined by the extent to which objectives are met and constraints are avoided. That makes preparing this statement one of the most critical steps in the risk management process. These are the things we must do and must avoid doing to succeed in solving the problems and attaining the opportunities we have identified. If we do not meet our objectives to at least some extent, our risk management activity has failed. If we violate our constraints, our risk management activity has failed.

The chain of logic is simple in best-practice risk management. If you meet your objectives and avoid your constraints, you will have solved your problems and attained your opportunities. Objectives and constraints provide a sound foundation for formulating and, later, evaluating risk management options.

So far, we are describing a rather broad and open risk management process. Not every risk management activity will require such breadth and openness. Some risk management activities are laser-focused on recurring issues of interest to only a few people. The process we are describing works as well for these activities as it does for public policy making. Risk management is a perfectly scalable process. Objectives, for an example, can be identified in 5 minutes, 5 hours, or 5 days.

### 3.3.2.3   Decide the need for a risk assessment

Your risk profile is complete, do you need a risk assessment or not? Not every risk management activity requires a risk assessment. Every risk management activity requires science-based evidence, but there will be times when there is enough evidence and knowledge in a room full of experts to know how to solve a well-defined problem. Other times, the risk profile will produce sufficient information to enable risk managers to know how to solve their problems and realize their opportunities.

When an issue requires immediate action or when a risk is well described by definitive data, a risk assessment will not be needed. If the risk managers already know what decision they are going to make, a sham assessment is not needed to justify a foregone decision. A relatively simple problem with little uncertainty, where the consequences of a wrong decision are minor, does not require a risk assessment. When the cars are speeding by, stay on the sidewalk. If the milk has turned sour, throw it way. Do not build in the floodplain. There are many instances where there is no need for a risk assessment. Then there will be times when the risk profile is insufficient for decision making.

### WHAT'S IN A RISK ASSESSMENT?

Want to start an argument? Go to a conference or listserv of risk people and ask the above question.

Risk assessment, like everything else about risk analysis, has many different definitions. A significant point of division for many seems to be whether risk assessment includes analysis that enables risk managers to evaluate the risks in addition to the analysis required to assess the risk. This could include, for example, benefit-cost analysis of risk management options. Some insist that such information is not and should not be part of risk assessment. They consider this risk management information that is used to evaluate the acceptability of an assessed risk or risk management option.

This narrow view may work for certain kinds of risk, like public health risks. But it falls apart for other kinds of risk like risks of financial or economic losses and gains. For our purposes, it is not so important where the necessary decision-making information is included as that it is included. So be aware that in some interpretations, risk assessment includes information from the natural sciences only, while in others, it may include much more extensive information.

A risk assessment can be useful when the data are not complete and there is much uncertainty or when there are multiple values in potential conflict. Risk assessments clarify the facts and are useful for issues of great concern to risk managers or stakeholders or when continuous decision making is in order. Risk assessment is sometimes used to guide research by identifying data gaps and significant uncertainties that need to be reduced. Assessments can establish a baseline estimate of a risk or examine the potential efficacy of new risk management options. They may be helpful in resolving international disputes. Practical issues that can affect the decision to do a risk assessment include:

- The time and resources available
- The urgency of a risk management response
- Consistency with responses to other similar issues
- The availability of scientific information

Deciding to do a risk assessment is a distinct result of the risk profiling task. A risk assessment should be requested when two conditions are met:

1. The risk profile fails to provide sufficient information for decision making.
2. The risk profile suggests there is sufficient information to complete a risk assessment.

Sometimes, there is so much uncertainty and such sparse data that it is not even feasible to attempt a risk assessment. In these situations, risk managers may make a preemptive decision based on caution or some other set of values. Alternatively, the risk profile results can be used to direct research toward filling the most critical data gaps so that risk assessment can then proceed. The decision of whether or not to do a risk assessment is often based on the results of the risk profile. That decision is the desired output of this activity. The remainder of this risk estimation discussion assumes that a risk assessment will be completed.

## REASONS FOR A RISK ASSESSMENT

- The information you have is not the information you want
- The information you want is not the information you need
- The information you need is not the information you can obtain
- The information you can obtain costs more than you want to pay

**Source: Adapted from Bernstein (1996)**

### 3.3.2.4   Request information needed

If the risk profile does not provide enough information to decide how to solve the problems or pursue the opportunities, risk managers must ask for the information they need to do so. They are going to need specific kinds of information in order to be able to meet their objectives and avoid their constraints, thereby solving the problems and attaining the opportunities. No one is better positioned to know what this information is than the person who will make those decisions, the risk manager.

Some of the information risk managers will need is likely to be scientific, evidence-based, factual information. This will be provided through risk assessment and possibly other evaluations like benefit-cost analysis and legal opinions. Some of the information they need will be more subjective in nature, for example, who is concerned with this issue and how do they feel about it? This will be obtained through other means, including a good public involvement or risk communication program.

It is absolutely essential, however, that risk managers explicitly ask for the information they know they are going to need to make a decision. It is not sufficient to issue a general request for a risk assessment based on a specific problem. Risk managers must ask risk assessors to answer specific questions in the risk assessment. If the managers do not ask the right question(s), they may not get the right information back from the risk assessment. Risk assessments that are not guided by questions to answer may produce information managers do not want to have, or they may fail to produce the information managers need to make a good decision.

## MY EXPERIENCE

I have worked on many risk management activities and risk assessments and I am often called in as a consultant, usually because things have not been going well. When it is my turn to speak, I hand out 3 × 5 index cards and ask everyone present to right down the question(s) they believe they are trying to answer through their risk assessment.

I then collect the cards and read them aloud. Amazingly, I have yet to have two cards identify the same question(s). How do we know what data to collect, what models to build, what analysis to do when we do not even agree on what question(s) we are trying to answer?

Getting the question(s) right is the next most critical step after problem identification.

The importance of the risk manager's questions can hardly be overstated. They guide the risk assessment and other evaluations required to provide the information necessary for decision making. Once these questions are answered, risk managers have the information they need to make decisions. These questions need to come from risk managers, often with input from assessors and stakeholders.

Risk analysis supports decision making by using science and evidence to identify what we know and what we do not know. It integrates this knowledge and uncertainty with social values to meet objectives and avoid constraints and thereby to solve problems. When the initial risk profile is completed, it is time to ask the most basic of all questions: "What do we know and what do we need to know?"

Risk managers ask questions. Risk assessors answer the risk questions. Other evaluations may answer other questions. If risk managers do not ask the right questions, the analysis that follows may well not meet decision makers' needs. These questions must be available at the start of a risk assessment. They must be specific and they should be specified or at least agreed by risk managers.

It is essential that they are written down. They are not real and concrete until one can articulate them in precise words on paper. The questions will almost surely be refined by negotiation among managers, assessors, and possibly stakeholders. The questions will evolve and change as our understanding of the problem and the decisions to be made evolve. Consequently, the questions must always be kept up to date and they must be known to everyone who is working on the risk assessment.

The desired output of this task is a written set of questions to be answered by the assessors and other analysts of the risk analysis team. Many risk assessment problems begin with missing, incomplete, inappropriate,

### SAMPLE QUESTIONS

How many annual cases of fluoroquinolone resistant Campylobacteriosis currently occur in the United States due to eating chicken?

How many annual cases of fluoroquinolone resistant Campylobacteriosis will occur in the United States in the future due to eating chicken if there are no changes in the current usage of fluoroquinolone drugs?

How many annual cases of fluoroquinolone resistant Campylobacteriosis will occur in the United States in the future due to eating chicken if the use of fluoroquinolone drugs in all food producing animals is prohibited?

How many annual cases of fluoroquinolone resistant Campylobacteriosis will occur in the United States in the future due to eating chicken if fluoroquinolone-treated chicken is sent for use in processed chicken products?

or just plain bad questions. To make sure they get the information they need to make a decision, risk managers need to ask for it directly.

An organization with a well-defined mission and recurring issues is likely to develop standard information needs for recurring problems. When those recurring information needs become general knowledge or a standard operating procedure (SOP), this task may be simpler for everyone because they know what to do and how to do it once the information needs are institutionalized. However, every organization faces enough unique situations that this task of getting the questions right should never be overlooked.

It is impossible to anticipate all the kinds of information risk managers may require for decision making early in the process. In general, four broad categories of questions can be anticipated. Risk managers will usually want to ask questions about how to:

1. Meet objectives and constraints
2. Characterize the risks of interest
3. Mitigate the risk
4. Address other values

Risk managers may require additional information in order to know how best to meet their objectives and avoid violating their constraints. How will you achieve/avoid them? How will you measure success toward them? What kinds of information do you need to have about them in order to achieve your objectives and avoid your constraints? Some questions can be expected to focus on these kinds of concerns. They can also overlap the other question categories.

Risk characterization questions are trickier to discuss at this point because the risk assessment steps have not yet been introduced, and this is one of them. For now, think of this as the step in the risk assessment where all the various bits of information are pulled together to characterize the likelihood and consequences of the various risks you are assessing. Risk managers must direct assessors to characterize risks in ways that are going to be of most use for decision making.

Suppose a risk to public health is caused by disease and the objective is to reduce the adverse human health effects of this disease. How should assessors characterize the risks? Do managers want to know the probability of contracting this disease for a given exposure? Is the exposure of interest an annual one or a lifetime one? Might it be more useful to have the numbers of people affected by the disease? If so, are managers interested in the numbers of infections, illnesses, hospitalizations, or deaths? Are there any special subpopulations of interest to managers? Risk managers need to take great pains to ask questions at the characterization level that, when answered, will give them the information they need to make a decision about whether and how to manage that risk.

It is wise to think of risk holistically when posing risk characterization questions. There may be separate questions about existing and future risks, residual risk, transferred risk, and transformed risk. A residual risk is the risk that remains after a risk management option is implemented. When a risk management option reduces risk at one point in time or space for one kind of event or activity while increasing risk at another time or space for the same event or activity, this is called a "transferred risk." When a risk management option alters the nature of a hazard, a population's exposure to that hazard, or the consequences of an exposure, this is called a "transformed risk." These concepts are not as readily applied to risks of uncertain potential gain.

Risk mitigation questions are another category of questions that will usually be appropriate to ask. What does a risk manager need to know to formulate and choose the best risk management option? What are others doing to manage this risk? What else can be done to manage this risk? How well are the different options likely to work? For example, how many illnesses will we have if there is a vaccination program? Specific questions about the efficacy of risk management options are important to ask.

Finally, there are, for lack of a better term, values questions. These focus on obvious values of importance that are not included in the objectives and constraints. Someone will almost always care about costs, benefits, environmental impacts, authority, legal considerations, and the like. Values questions may also include stakeholders' concerns and their perceptions.

Once the questions are prepared, assessors and managers need to discuss them and what they mean. When a risk manager asks, "What is the risk of getting ill by eating an egg?" you may need to parse the question. What is meant by an egg? What kind of egg? Must it be in a shell or can it be processed? What do you mean by ill? How ill and for how long? A question that is perfectly clear to one person may be a complete mystery to another. Communication between managers and assessors is necessary to gain a clear common understanding of the questions. It may be necessary to negotiate the list of questions at times. Some questions may be incomplete, unreasonable, or impossible to answer. When that happens, risk assessors must tell the risk manager. If important questions are missing, they should be added. Expect questions to be clarified, modified, deleted, and added to throughout the risk management activity.

As mentioned previously, not all questions are science questions. It may take more than a risk assessment to answer all of the risk manager's questions. Some activities may require legal analysis, benefit-cost analysis, consumer surveys, market assessment, and the like and these kinds of analyses may be considered outside the purview of risk assessment in some circumstances.

At this point, we are up to three important pieces of paper that are essential to the successful completion of the risk management activity. They are:

- A problems and opportunities statement
- An objectives and constraints statement
- A list of questions the risk manager would like answered

If you vet the contents of these three pieces of paper with your stakeholders, you have the beginnings of an excellent risk communication process. These three pieces of paper and the process you went through to prepare them also provide an excellent basis for the eventual documentation of your risk management activity.

### 3.3.2.5   Initiate the risk assessment

With a decision to do a risk assessment in one hand and the questions to be answered by the assessment in the other, it is time to initiate the risk assessment. It is the risk manager's responsibility to provide the resources necessary to get the risk assessment done. In general, that means assembling an appropriate team of experts to carry out the task, providing them with sufficient time, budget, and other necessary resources, and interacting with them extensively enough to instruct them clearly on the information needed for decision making. All of this is to take place while maintaining a functional separation between risk assessment and risk management activities.

---

**FUNCTIONAL SEPARATION**

Functional separation means separating the tasks carried out as part of risk assessment from those carried out by risk management at the time they are performed. Some organizations may have separate offices to conduct the two tasks. In some situations, the same individual(s) may be responsible for management and assessment. This occurs most often in resource poor situations, but it may also occur with routine and simple issues.

It is important that safeguards be in place to ensure that management and assessment tasks are carried out separately of each other, even if they are performed by the same individuals. Management and assessment are fundamentally different. The objective assessment needs to remain objective and the subjective judgment needs to remain apart from it.

An independent interdisciplinary team of scientists, analysts, and other experts is preferred for conducting risk assessment. In routine situations, in-house experts and personnel are sufficient for a risk assessment team. In more structured or international environments, risk assessments may be carried out by an independent scientific institution, an expert group attached to an institution, or an expert group assembled for the express purposes of the risk assessment.

Risk managers are responsible for supporting the work of the risk assessment team and other evaluations by ensuring that they have the necessary resources. In general, a good risk assessment policy will have established guidelines for much of this administrative work on a once-and-for-all basis before the actual risk assessment is initiated. The roles and responsibilities of key personnel, the manner in which different organizational units interact, milestones, methods for communicating and coordinating—all of these administrative matters are the responsibility of the risk managers.

### 3.3.2.6 Consider the results of the risk assessment

After initiating the risk assessment, assessors go off and complete their work in a risk assessment, which is the subject of the next chapter. When the risk assessment is completed and submitted to the risk manager, the major question at this step in the risk management process is: "Did risk managers get answers to their questions that they can use for decision making?"

---

**EXAMPLE OF RISK ASSESSMENT ROLES**

The FDA's Center for Food Safety and Applied Nutrition has established three unique positions to help with consistency, coordination, and making risk decisions. They are:

- Science Advisor for Risk Analysis
- Risk Analysis Coordinator
- Risk Assessment Project Manager

---

The risk assessment should clearly and completely answer the questions asked by the risk managers to the greatest extent possible. Those answers should identify and quantify sources of instrumental uncertainties in risk estimates and in the answers provided to risk managers. Whenever the uncertainty might affect the answer to a critical question and, consequently, the risk manager's decision, or decision outcomes, this information must be effectively communicated. Hence, in addition to getting answers to their questions, risk managers must also know the strengths and weaknesses of the risk assessment and its outputs. Chapter 7 is devoted to practical approaches to decision making under uncertainty.

It is not necessary for the risk managers to understand all the details of the risk assessment, but they must be sufficiently familiar with the risk assessment techniques and models used to be able to explain them and the assessment results to external stakeholders. To understand the weaknesses and limitations of the risk assessment, it is important to:

- Understand the nature, sources, and extent of instrumental knowledge uncertainty and natural variability in risk estimates.
- Understand how the answers to critical questions might be changed or how decision outcomes might vary as a result of this uncertainty.
- Be aware of all important assumptions made during the risk assessment as well as their impact on the results of the assessment and the answers to the questions and the range of decision outcomes.
- Peer review may be a useful tool for discovering implicit assumptions of the risk assessment and other instrumental uncertainties that may have escaped the assessors' awareness.
- Identify research needs to fill the key data gaps in scientific knowledge to improve the results of the risk assessment in future iterations.

If the assessment has adequately met the information needs of the risk manager, it is complete. If the assessment has failed to provide the necessary information for any reason, another iteration of the assessment may be in order.

## 3.4   Risk evaluation

The risk assessment is now complete and it is time to evaluate the risk following the steps shown in Figure 3.4. Is the risk acceptable? This is the first significant decision for the risk manager to make. It requires the risk manager to be able to distinguish two important ideas: acceptable risk and tolerable risk. An acceptable risk is a risk whose probability of occurrence is so small or whose consequences are so slight or whose benefits (perceived or real) are so great that individuals or groups in society are willing to take or be subjected to the risk that the event might occur. An acceptable risk requires no risk management; it is, by definition, acceptable. A risk that is not acceptable is, therefore, unacceptable and by definition must be managed.

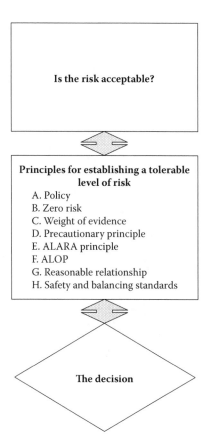

*Figure 3.4* Risk evaluation steps.

It is conceptually possible to take steps to reduce an unacceptable level of risk to an acceptable level. More often than not, however, unacceptable risks are managed to tolerable levels. A tolerable risk is a nonnegligible risk that has not yet been reduced to an acceptable level, think of it as a subset of unacceptable risk. The risk is tolerated for one of three reasons. We may be unable to reduce the risk further; the costs of doing so are considered excessive; or the magnitude of the benefits associated with the risky activity are too great to reduce it further. A tolerable risk is not an acceptable risk, but its severity has been reduced to a point where it is tolerated.

If a risk is initially judged to be unacceptable, risk managers will seek to determine a level of risk that can be tolerated if the risk cannot be reduced to an acceptable level. Several principles (see Figure 3.4) have been

## OPPORTUNITIES FOR GAIN

What is an acceptable uncertain potential gain? Does it make sense to talk about a tolerable level of such risk? It is impossible to anticipate every potential gain situation but, for a vast majority of them, the concepts of acceptable and tolerable risk hold up pretty well.

Let us consider the potential for economic gain as the endpoint. Acceptability is going to be defined by both the consequence, for example a net negative or net positive outcome, and its probability. A low probability of a large positive outcome may be acceptable while a high probability of a small positive outcome may not be, or vice versa. In situations where the combination of consequence and its probability are not acceptable, in a desirable sense, the risk can be managed to the point that it becomes tolerable. This is done by taking steps to increase the likelihood of a desirable outcome or by increasing the magnitude of the potential beneficial consequences.

Risk taking is essentially different from risk avoiding. Risk-taking decisions are conscious decisions to expose one's self to a risk that could have otherwise been avoided. Consequently, managing uncertainty prior to decision making or during evolutionary decision making is a significant risk management strategy for opportunity risks.

used to determine a tolerable level of risk (TLR). Once a methodology for establishing the TLR is chosen, it is the risk manager's responsibility to determine the TLR as part of the risk evaluation activities. Very often, for example, the TLR is less an explicit determination than it is a default result of what it is possible to do. This determination overlaps considerably with subsequent risk control activities.

Bear in mind that risk managers are not, at this point, being asked to evaluate the effectiveness of any specific risk management options that may have been assessed in the risk assessment. That particular evaluation task is considered later under the risk control activities. It is also helpful to bear in mind that we are describing an iterative process in what amounts to a linear narrative. It will often be necessary to double back on the process and repeat a few steps. So, although the description here might suggest that the risk and all risk management options are assessed in a risk assessment that is then handed, complete, to risk managers, the real process is not always so simple.

**INPUT AND FEEDBACK**

Determining what risk is acceptable and establishing a tolerable level of risk (TLR) for risks that are unacceptable are decisions that cannot often be made without input from stakeholders and the public. In some decision contexts, this may require a rather extensive public involvement program. In others, it may be a simple risk communication task. Offering opportunities for input and providing feedback on views about what is acceptable, unacceptable, and tolerable is a critical part of an effective risk communication program.

Determining whether a risk is acceptable or not is a matter of subjective judgment. It is not a scientific determination. There is potential for the uncertainty about the best decision to make to increase at this point if the risk manager's information does not include the views of key stakeholders or if the risk communication program has not yet provided these stakeholders with opportunities for input and feedback. It is usually important to understand the risk attitudes of key stakeholders when establishing a TLR. The principles described in the following section can be used to help determine whether the assessed risk is acceptable or not. They can also be used to find a TLR when the risk is unacceptable.

## 3.4.1  Principles for establishing acceptable and tolerable levels of risk

There is no magic bullet to be found in this section. Deciding whether an assessed risk is acceptable or not and determining a tolerable level of risk for risks that cannot be rendered acceptable are fundamentally searches for subjective targets. Does the risk manager seek the highest possible level of protection, a desirable level of protection, an achievable level of protection, or something that is practical (implementable) or affordable? Does equity matter? Must there be a consistent level of protection, or is the economic efficiency of a level of protection more important? There is no one answer that will satisfy everyone. Therefore, the process by which this decision is reached may be as important as the decision rule that is used to reach it. To determine an acceptable or tolerable level of risk, managers must take into account the scientific evidence, the uncertainty, and the values evident in their objectives and constraints. Several principles used by risk managers are reviewed here briefly.

### 3.4.1.1   Policy

Some decisions have already been made for the risk manager by persons higher in the decision-making hierarchy. These may be the owners of a company, upper management, Congress, the president, or other elected officials. In the United States, for example, Congress and the president may pass authorizing legislation that prescribes what an agency can and must do. In that case, the risk manager's job is to figure out the best way to do it.

---

**THE DELANEY CLAUSE**

The Delaney clause is a part of the 1958 Food Additives Amendment (section 409) to the 1954 Federal Food, Drug, and Cosmetic Act (FFDCA). This clause governs regulation of pesticide residues in processed foods. It establishes that no residues from pesticides found to cause cancer in animals will be allowed as a food additive. This means that tolerance levels must be based only on the risk of carcinogenicity and that the benefits of the pesticide may not be considered. This clause was considered, at the time, to have set a zero-risk standard.

---

Some risk issues may be resolved by a court decision. Decision contexts initiated as a result of administrative or other legal proceedings are often circumscribed by the entity that orders the decision action. Courts at all levels of jurisdiction are increasingly being drawn into policy decisions that could affect the principles for determining an acceptable or tolerable risk.

Decisions made in the public sector, especially by agencies and organizations acting as stewards of a public asset or trust, will often be constrained by policy. Working with a government agency often means dealing with their policy restrictions and requirements. International treaties and agreements may also identify solutions or limit options. In the private sector, acceptable and tolerable levels of risk may be established in an entity's risk appetite or risk tolerance, which are topics discussed in Chapter 6.

### 3.4.1.2   Zero risk

Banning risky activities has been a popular approach in years gone by. Making actions that involve any risk at all taboo and declaring them forbidden has been tried in the past when it was once possible to imagine zero risk. Years ago, the limits of our knowledge and of scientific detection made it possible to find comfort in laws that appeared to legislate safety as a matter of zero risk. See the Delaney clause text box for an example.

By the middle of the 1980s, decision makers began to abandon the notion of zero risk in favor of more realistic versions of negligible risk. The one-in-a-million standard seems to have captured our imagination early. This evolved from and morphed into a notion of de minimis risk, a numerical value of risk too small to be bothered about. You can think of negligible and de minimis as "practically zero" without doing any real damage to the concepts.

Society and policy makers have, by and large, abandoned the idea that zero risk is a realistic measure of acceptable risk. Establishing a level of de minimis risk remains a viable concept for determining acceptable and tolerable levels of risk in certain settings.

### DE MINIMIS RISK

A careful reading of official documents about the de minimis principle, as well as of relevant journal articles, shows that it is usually explained along one of the following three formulations. The specific-number view says a risk is de minimis provided its probability falls below a certain number, for example, $10^{-6}$. The nondetectability view says a risk is de minimis provided it cannot be scientifically established whether the risk has in fact materialized or not. The natural-occurrence view for an anthropogenic risk says a risk is de minimis provided its anthropogenic risk does not exceed the natural occurrence of this type of risk.

**Source: Peterson (2002)**

### 3.4.1.3   Weight of evidence

We tend to like once-and-for-all resolution of problems on the basis of compelling scientific evidence. In an uncertain world, the truth is not always easy to see. Data gaps and conflicting evidence often obfuscate risk management decisions. In a weight-of-evidence approach to evaluating risk, risk managers assess the credibility of conflicting evidence about hazards and risks in a systematic and objective manner. A formal weight-of-evidence process may rely on a diverse group of scientists to examine the evidence to reach consensus views. The evidence must be of sufficient strength, coherence, and consistency to support an inference that a hazard and a risk exist.

Evaluating the weight of evidence is an ongoing activity that attempts to balance positive and negative evidence of harmful effects based on relevant data. Thus, the evaluation of risk is conditional on the available evidence and subject to change as new evidence becomes available. When there is uncertainty about the nature of a risk, a weight-of-evidence approach may be useful in establishing whether it is acceptable or tolerable.

### 3.4.1.4  Precautionary principle

Precaution may be described in this context as refraining from action if the consequences of the action are not well understood. It is prudent avoidance. The precautionary principle is broadly based on the notion that human and ecological health are irreplaceable human goods. Their protection should be treated as the paramount concern for regulatory organizations and government. All other concerns are secondary.

The precautionary principle is controversial and heavily influenced by culture and uncertainty. In a very loose and informal sense, the precautionary principle suggests that when there is significant uncertainty about a significant risk, we should err on the side of precaution, if we are to err at all. That means that activities that could give rise to catastrophic outcomes should be prohibited. It also means that if inaction could give rise to catastrophic outcomes, we should act, not wait. The precautionary principle is generally considered to be most appropriate in the early stages of an unfolding risk problem, when the potential for serious or irreversible health consequences is great, or when the likelihood of occurrence or magnitude of consequence is highly uncertain. The desire for precaution is usually positively related to the amount of uncertainty in a decision problem. The precautionary principle can be invoked for decision making when uncertainties are large or intractable.

---

### WINGSPREAD STATEMENT

When an activity raises threats of harm to human health or the environment, precautionary measures should be taken even if some cause and effect relationships are not fully established scientifically. In this context the proponent of an activity, rather than the public, should bear the burden of proof. The process of applying the precautionary principle must be open, informed and democratic and must include potentially affected parties. It must also involve an examination of the full range of alternatives, including no action.

**Source: Wingspread Conference, January, 1998**

### 3.4.1.5 ALARA principle

ALARA is an acronym for As Low As Reasonably Achievable. Technology and cost present two realistic constraints on what it is possible to achieve in terms of risk reduction. If a risk is not yet as low as is reasonably achievable, it is unacceptable according to this principle. One popular criterion for establishing a tolerable level of risk is to get risk as low as we are capable of making it. Then what choice do we have but to tolerate the risk that remains?

Sometimes the ALARA principle is used to take risks even lower than an acceptable level of risk. Minimizing risks even below levels that would be acceptable is sometimes justified based on the presumption that what constitutes "acceptable risk" can vary widely among individuals.

Best available technology (BAT) is a related concept. It differs in a potentially significant way, however, as BAT says to use the best available with no further qualification. ALARA introduces the idea of reasonableness, and this opens the management door to the consideration of other factors like cost and social acceptability. BAT does not consider these other factors.

### 3.4.1.6 Appropriate level of protection

An appropriate level of protection (ALOP) defines or is defined by the risk society is willing to tolerate. Despite the promising sound of this principle, it is little more than circular reasoning because it presumes one has found a way to identify the holy grail of what is "appropriate" for society. In fact, it is often little more than a statement of the degree of protection that is to be achieved by the risk management option implemented. Policy (see text box) or a rigorous public involvement program provide alternative ways to define the ALOP.

The significant contribution of this concept is that it flips the focus from risk to protection, where we might think of protection as akin to different degrees of safety. The factors used to determine an ALOP typically include:

- Technical feasibility of prevention and control options
- Risks that may arise from risk management interventions
- Magnitude of benefits of a risky activity and the availability of substitute activities
- Cost of prevention and control versus effectiveness of risk reduction
- Public risk reduction preferences, that is, public values
- Distribution of risks and benefits

**ALOP EXAMPLE**

The commitment of FDA, FSIS, and CDC to reduce foodborne listeriosis was formally reaffirmed as a national public health goal in the Healthy People 2010 initiative coordinated by the United States Department of Health and Human Services (US DHHS). The federal government established a goal of working with industry, public health, and research communities to achieve an additional 50% reduction in listeriosis by 2010.

**Source: FDA (2003b)**

### 3.4.1.7   Reasonable relationship

This principle suggests that costs of risk management should bear "a reasonable relationship" to the corresponding reductions in risks. It is not a benefit-cost analysis but it is an attempt to balance nonmonetary benefits (i.e., risk management outputs and outcomes) and the monetary costs of achieving them. Cost-effectiveness and incremental cost analysis are often used as the basis for determining the reasonableness of this relationship.

### 3.4.1.8   Safety and balancing standards

Safety maintains deep roots within the risk analysis paradigm. A great many safety standards have been used to establish the tolerable level of risk. Safety standards encompass a bundle of standard-setting methods that rely ultimately on some degree of subjective judgment. For example, the zero-risk standard mentioned previously is one possible safety standard. Zero just happens to be one of many potential thresholds that can be established to define safety. Any nonzero level of risk can be stipulated as safe, acceptable, or tolerable. In fact, TLR has been dangled as one such tantalizing threshold standard in some of the literature. If we could develop a TLR for dam safety or for food safety or for transportation modalities, policy making would be much easier.

Many determinations of a TLR require a subjective balancing decision. Risks of uncertain potential gain or benefits may be best served by using some type of balancing standard. For example, risk-benefit trade-off analysis generally implies that greater benefits mean we are willing to accept a greater level of risk in exchange for those benefits. The risk-benefit trade-off may explain why we are all willing to assume the risk of driving in a modern society.

Comparative risk analysis (CRA) ranks risks for the seriousness of the threat they pose. It began as an environmental decision-making tool (USAID, 1990, 1993a, 1993b, 1994; EPA, 1985, 1992a, 1992b, 1994; World Bank, 1994) used to systematically measure, compare, and rank environmental problems or issues. It typically results in a list of issues or activities ranked in terms of relative risks. The most common purpose of comparative risk analysis is to establish priorities for a government agency. The concept is perfectly adaptable to any organization.

Benefit-cost analysis is another kind of balancing standard used to determine what is acceptable or tolerable by attempting to identify and express the advantages and disadvantages of a risk or risk management option in dollar terms. It is considered a useful measure of economic efficiency.

In addition to threshold and balancing standards, procedural standards are sometimes used to define what is acceptable or tolerable. Procedural standards typically identify an agreed-upon process, which is often the result of negotiation or a referendum of some sort. If the agreed-upon process is followed, then the results of that process are considered acceptable or at least tolerable.

## 3.4.2  The decision

If the assessed risk is judged by any one of these or any other method to be acceptable, there is little more for the risk manager to do. However, an unacceptable risk must be managed. The ideal would be to manage it to an acceptable level, and when that cannot be done it should be managed to a tolerable level. There are six broad strategies for managing risk. These are:

1. Risk taking
2. Risk avoidance
3. Reduce the probability of the risk event (prevent) and increase the probability of a potential gain (enhance)
4. Reduce the consequence of the risk event (mitigate) and increase the consequence of a potential gain (intensify)
5. Risk pooling and sharing
6. Retain the risk

Risk managers may choose to take a risk when it presents an opportunity for gain that is acceptable or at least tolerable. When it comes to losses with no chance of gain, it is usually preferable to avoid such a risk whenever possible. If avoidance is not practical, we can try to manage either or both of the two dimensions of risk. Risk prevention reduces the likelihood of exposure to a hazard or otherwise reduces the probability

## NO ONE SPEAKS THIS CAREFULLY

Beware. I have gone to some effort to try to carefully differentiate risk management strategies in the text. In my experience, no one speaks quite this carefully. In fact, mitigation, management, control, treatment, avoidance, prevention, and probably several other terms are all used interchangeably. So, if you take pains to speak carefully and precisely, do not assume others hear you with the same precision. Take the time to clarify your meanings.

of an undesirable outcome. Conversely, efforts can be made to increase the likelihood of gain from an opportunity risk. This is an enhancement strategy.

Risk mitigation allows that risky events will occur, so it seeks to reduce the impact of the risk by reducing the consequences of the event. Increasing the magnitude of a potential positive consequence, intensification, is another opportunity risk management strategy. A fifth option is to pool the risks into a larger group and share these risks over a greater spatial or temporal extent. A sixth strategy is to retain the risk. When no viable option for managing the risk can be found, we have no option but to put up with the risk as is. As this does nothing to lessen the risk or its impacts, some would not call it a strategy for managing risk.

If the risk manager's role in the risk assessment can be described as a positive one, then the manager's role shifts to a normative one in these risk evaluation tasks. Here, the risk manager describes the world as it "ought" to be. This is a subjective deliberative decision. This normative role continues into the manager's risk control responsibilities.

## 3.5   Risk control

Presuming the risk has been judged to be unacceptable during risk evaluation, the risk manager's job now becomes reducing the risk to an acceptable or tolerable level. Risk control is a term of art used to avoid greater confusion with the risk management strategies described previously. It may be misleading to suggest that we can control some risks. It may be more honest to say that we struggle to manage them. However, calling this risk management activity "risk management" might cause even greater confusion. So be forewarned not to interpret control too literally in the current context, risk treatment is a synonym. The basic tasks during this risk control phase of the manager's job are shown in Figure 3.5.

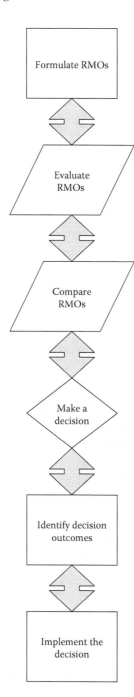

*Figure 3.5* Risk control steps.

The extent to which the public and stakeholders are engaged in this phase may show the greatest range of variation of any risk management activity. Private risk management decisions may not involve anyone outside the organization. Collective decision-making processes can involve extensive public involvement programs for the risk control activities.

## 3.5.1  Formulating risk management options

What does success look like? Risk management options (RMOs) are strategies that describe specific ways your risk management objectives can be achieved. These strategies are subordinate to your objectives. An RMO is relevant only to the extent that it helps you meet your objectives. Best-practice risk management recognizes that objectives can be achieved in a variety of ways and formulates alternative strategies that reflect these different ways.

---

### THE PROBLEM IS WE NEED A LEVEE

Many problems are initially identified in terms of a solution. Risk analysis focuses on getting the problem right. The problem may be flooding, it may be unrestricted land development or any other number of things. A levee is one possible solution. It is common for many problem-solving processes to begin with someone identifying the solution before the problem is clearly identified. Keep track of and consider that solution but do not let it prevent you from identifying alternative means of achieving your objectives or from properly identifying the problem.

---

Laws, authorities, policies, budget priorities, and politics may limit what you can actually do. None of these should limit the things you think, however. Formulate RMOs comprehensively and creatively without respect to any limitations. Thinking creatively and comprehensively about solutions to risk problems is one area in which there is room for substantial improvement for many organizations. Getting risk managers to consider a broad array of risk management options has not been the easiest thing to do. One major reason for this is that we tend to favor solutions we are familiar with or that we have the authority and ability to act upon. There is a certain obvious appeal to this sort of thinking.

If there is an effective way to manage a risk that your organization cannot implement, others may implement it voluntarily if the idea is good enough. Or perhaps there are ways to motivate those who can implement a good idea to do so. Bear in mind that good ideas for achieving worthy objectives are valid reasons for organizations to be granted new authorities.

RMOs may be formulated by the risk analysis team with input from stakeholders and decision makers. They may be imposed from above by higher authorities. They may be suggestions from the public or new scientific or technological developments. The ideas can come from Congress, agency staff, industry, government officials at all levels, academia, "the public," television, science fiction, your left frontal lobe, or a bottle of beer. They are the children of perspiration, inspiration, and imitation. An RMO may be proposed at any point in the risk management process. Some processes may begin because someone has framed a problem (incorrectly, I hasten to add) in terms of a solution.

The process of identifying RMOs is simplified by considering a few option formulation steps. If risk managers have done a good job identifying objectives and constraints, the simplest way to begin is to identify measures that could achieve each objective. A measure is a feature that constitutes part of a strategy or RMO. Think of a feature as some physical change or an activity, where an activity is a change in the way we do something. So, for objective 1, we identify as many measures that could contribute to this objective as possible, then repeat this process for each objective and constraint.

Second, you formulate or construct RMOs from these measures. Think of the measures as building blocks and RMOs as the "structures" you build to solve problems and attain opportunities.

The third step is to reformulate RMOs. Like the rest of the risk management process, RMO formulation is iterative. Once an option is formulated, see if you can refine it. When evaluation of the options begins, it can be very effective to reformulate or tweak the options to improve their performance.

### KEY POINT

When developing RMOs, quantity counts more than quality in the initial stages. You cannot be sure you have the best option unless you have considered many options. Avoid the temptation to fall in love with your first idea. Formulating alternative RMOs is an essential step in good risk management.

How do you know when a set of measures is an RMO? A good RMO should be complete, effective, efficient, and acceptable. Completeness means all the necessary pieces are accounted for and included in the option. Effectiveness means the mix of measures meets the objectives as well as possible and avoids violating constraints as much as possible. Efficiency means there is no less costly option that produces the same benefits and benefits cannot be increased without increasing costs. Neither can adverse effects be decreased without decreasing benefits or increasing costs. Acceptability means no laws or regulations are violated and there is no evident reason why the RMO could not be implemented.

## 3.5.2   Evaluating risk management options

Earlier, we spoke of evaluating the risks that are assessed in the risk assessment. Don't confuse that with evaluating the risk management options that are being considered for use in managing unacceptable risks to a tolerable level. In some cases, the performance of these RMOs may have been assessed simultaneously with the risks themselves in the risk assessment. In other situations, RMOs will not even be identified until after the risk assessment is completed. The actual sequence of events can vary with the nature of the risk and the available information in any given decision context.

No matter which sequence your own risk management activity might follow, there comes a time when the formulation of RMOs is complete enough that you need to begin to evaluate these ideas. This is part of the nonscientific work of the risk management process. Values, beliefs, and biases all enter the process here, and appropriately so. This is where risk managers begin to weigh their decision options and earn their pay.

After RMOs have been comprehensively formulated, to get from a number of options to the best option you must:

- Evaluate options
- Compare options
- Make a decision (select the best option)

These can be discrete steps or they may be all mixed together. Like other risk management responsibilities, these can be iterative tasks. Up until now, the emphasis has been on generating as many serviceable ideas for managing an unacceptable risk as are possible. Only now do we begin to go through those ideas and evaluate them to judge which are viable solutions and which are not.

Evaluation of RMOs is a deliberative analytical process. Evaluation and comparison require measurements of evaluation and comparison criteria. These will be produced by risk assessors and other analysts at the direction of risk managers. In evaluation, risk managers look at each RMO individually and considers it on its own merits. Think of this evaluation step as a pass/fail decision that qualifies some options for serious consideration

*Table 3.1* Evaluating an RMO via comparison scenarios without additional risk management and with additional risk management

| Effect | Future without | Future with | Change |
|---|---|---|---|
| Annual illnesses | 50,000 | 20,000 | –30,000 |
| Cost | $0 | $150 million | +$150 million |
| Benefits | Unchanged | Reduced | Decrease |
| Jobs | Unchanged | Lose 2,000 | –2,000 |

for implementation as a solution and rejects others. One of the simplest ways to evaluate an RMO is to examine the effects it would have on the risk management objectives and constraints. The underlying presumption, once again, is that if we achieve our objectives and avoid violating the constraints, we will solve our problems and realize our opportunities. That is our definition of a successful risk management process.

It is, of course, common practice to focus carefully on the management of risks during the evaluation process. In a good risk management process, risk reduction can be expected to be prominently displayed among the risk management objectives.

The effects of an RMO can be identified by comparing two scenarios as shown in Table 3.1. Identifying the existing levels of risk, also known as inherent risk, defines one scenario. Reestimating those risk levels with an RMO in place and functioning, that is, residual risk, is the second scenario. The differences between these scenarios can be attributed to the efficacy of the RMO, all other things being equal. Table 3.1 shows a hypothetical evaluation using a scenario without any additional risk management activity (without) and a scenario with a new RMO in place (with) as the basis for the evaluation.

There are currently 50,000 illnesses and implementing RMO 1 will reduce that total to 20,000. The change is a reduction of 30,000 illnesses. The changes are what the risk managers will evaluate. If the objectives and constraints were to reduce adverse health effects, minimize costs, and avoid reductions in benefits and job losses, then a subjective judgment needs to be made about whether this particular option does this in a manner satisfactory enough to warrant serious consideration for implementation as a solution. The process is repeated for each individual RMO. All scenario comparisons would use the same "without" condition scenario as the starting point. The "with" condition scenario will vary from one RMO to another.

Uncertainties affecting estimates of the evaluation criteria must be considered at this step. For simplicity, the values presented in Table 3.1 are shown as point estimates. In actual fact they may be probabilistic estimates reflecting varying degrees of natural variability and knowledge uncertainty.

Note that an option is not being compared to other options at this point. We are simply separating our RMOs into two piles. One pile "qualifies" for serious consideration for implementation and the other pile does not. The reject pile can either be reformulated to improve their performance or dropped from further consideration. The qualified RMOs will later be compared to one another.

Evaluation requires evaluation criteria. The risk management objectives and constraints are a logical source of such criteria, but risk managers are free to evaluate on any basis that serves their decision-making needs. At times, the evaluation criteria may be a subset of the objectives and constraints or a set of criteria quite different from them. The risk manager's role in evaluation includes identifying evaluation criteria and selecting qualified plans. The selection of these plans for further consideration is sometimes delegated to the assessors, as this is a screening decision. Assessors analyze the RMO's contributions to the evaluation criteria for the managers.

### 3.5.2.1   Comparison methods

Evaluating plans requires a comparison of evaluation criteria values with and without an RMO in place. To generate estimates of the effects of an RMO, some sort of comparison method is required. There are at least three different ways to compare scenarios: gap analysis, before-and-after comparison, and with-and-without comparison. The latter is generally preferred as the most objective comparison, and it is recommended for generating measurements for evaluating the impacts of an RMO. The three methods are shown in Figure 3.6 and described below. This comparison of evaluation criteria for a specific RMO is distinct and different from the comparison of alternative RMOs.

An evaluation criterion can be anything relevant to risk managers for this task. A common first step in evaluation is to describe the baseline

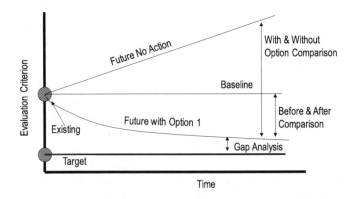

*Figure 3.6* Three methods for comparing scenarios.

condition of this criterion estimate. The baseline measure is often assumed to be the existing level of the criterion over time with no change. The "without" condition describes the most likely future condition of the evaluation criterion in the absence of any intentional change in risk management. This scenario shows the future criterion values without additional risk management. Every RMO is to be evaluated against this same "without" condition to estimate its effect on the criterion.

The "with" condition describes the most likely future condition of the evaluation criteria with a specific RMO in place. Each intervention (e.g., RMO 1) has its own unique "with" condition. Therefore, RMO 1 will have a different "with" condition than RMO 2, and so on.

The best evaluation method compares the "with" and "without" condition levels of the evaluation criteria for each RMO. The resulting analysis provides values like those shown in Table 3.1. These values serve as the basis for qualifying an RMO for further consideration or not.

Note that the before-and-after comparison, popularized by the National Environmental Policy Act (NEPA) process and also quite common in the food safety and some public health fields, could yield significantly different insights about the efficacy of an RMO. There are several definitions of gap analysis. Here, gap analysis refers to the difference between a prescribed target level of a criterion (or other effect) and what you are able to attain in reality. This graphic represents a hypothetical example to illustrate the concept; other trends in the scenarios are possible.

### 3.5.3 Comparing risk management options

A good RMO formulation process will produce numerous alternative solutions to a problem. A successful evaluation process will identify several of these as viable solutions. At this point, it is necessary to compare the qualified solutions to identify the best one from among them. Comparison is an analytical step. It means establishing the similarities and dissimilarities among RMOs and contrasting the merits among them. Making a decision is based on weighing the differences among the compared RMOs such as those shown in Table 3.2.

A good comparison process identifies differences among the RMOs that matter to people. It also makes the trade-offs among the options clear. A simplified example of a comparison summary is shown in Table 3.2. For simplicity, it ignores the complication of expressing uncertainty about these estimates. It is important to understand that uncertainty may be an essential part of an actual comparison. Each column represents a risk management option that has been qualified by the evaluation process. The rows represent decision criteria that have been identified as important to decision makers.

*Table 3.2* Comparing RMOs by contrasting the differences in their effects
on decision criteria

| Effect | RMO1 | RMO2 | RMO3 |
|---|---|---|---|
| Annual illnesses | −30,000 | −40,000 | −10,000 |
| Illnesses remaining | 20,000 | 10,000 | 40,000 |
| Cost | +$150 million | +$500 million | +$100 million |
| Benefits | Decrease | Decrease | No change |
| Jobs | −2,000 | 0 | −500 |

Table 3.2 shows how different RMOs make different contributions to
the risk management objectives (assuming, for convenience, that they are
reflected in the criteria chosen). RMO 2 reduces the number of illnesses
more than any other option does. It also costs more. A summary table like
this enables decision makers to see the differences among the options, and
it makes the trade-offs more evident. Again, you are cautioned that these
determinations are more difficult to make when the uncertainties in these
estimates are reflected. Methods for doing this are discussed in later chapters.

Risk managers will direct the comparison process, although they will
not usually do the supporting analysis. A critical management step is
identifying the criteria to be used in the comparison. It is not unusual for
risk assessors to suggest criteria and their metrics in unique situations. The
comparison provides the analytical summary of the information that will
form the foundation for a final decision. Thus, the risk manager's main role
in comparison is often to request and understand the information that will
be used to make a decision.

Comparisons are easiest when all effects can be reduced to a single,
common metric. This, conceptually, could be lives saved, illnesses
prevented, jobs created, or any metric at all. In benefit-cost analysis, that
common metric is monetary. Many, if not most, comparisons involve
incommensurable metrics. These situations will involve trade-off
techniques. Those techniques can range from simple ad hoc decisions to
sophisticated multicriteria decision analysis techniques. An example of
the latter follows.

### 3.5.3.1 *Multicriteria decision analysis*
A decision is always easier to make when you consider only one
dimension of the problem and when you are the only decision maker.
Risk management decisions, however, are often complex and multifaceted.
They can involve many risk managers, each with a different responsibility
for the RMO, as well as stakeholders with different values, and priorities.
They often involve complex trade-offs of risks, benefits, costs, social values,
and other impacts because of the values in conflict as a result of the many

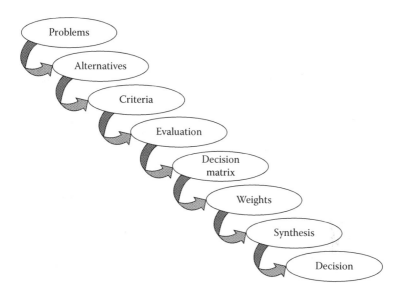

*Figure 3.7* MCDA process.

perspectives represented by the stakeholders to a decision. One of the most predictable sources of uncertainty in any public decision-making process and in many private ones is what importance or weights should be assigned to the decision criteria. Multicriteria decision analysis (MCDA) is a bundle of techniques and methodologies that enables analysts to reduce the varied effects of different RMOs to a single utility metric that enables more direct comparison. Figure 3.7 shows the steps in a typical MCDA process (Yoe, 2002). Through the evaluation step in the figure, this process tracks closely with the risk management process described here. What MCDA adds is a useful methodology for comparing options.

Multicriteria decision problems generally involve choosing one of a number of alternative solutions to a problem based on how well those alternatives rate against a set of decision criteria. The criteria themselves are weighted in terms of their relative importance to the decision makers. The overall "score" of an alternative is the weighted sum of its ratings against all criteria. The ultimate value of MCDA, both as a tool and a process, is that it helps us to identify and understand conflicts and the trade-offs they involve.

A risk management activity defines the problem and, done well, fits the MCDA process neatly. It provides alternative means to solve the problem. Decision criteria are identified, quite possibly, from the objectives and constraints during the evaluation and comparison processes. The last four steps of a generic MCDA process are often executed by a variety of user-friendly software tools.

Choose Best Risk Management Option
Annual Illnesses Reduced
Benefits
Cost ($ Millions)
Jobs Lost
Alternatives
RMO1
RMO2
RMO3

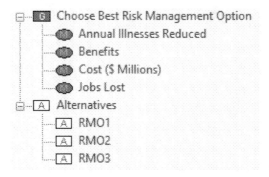

*Figure 3.8* A simple MCDA model.

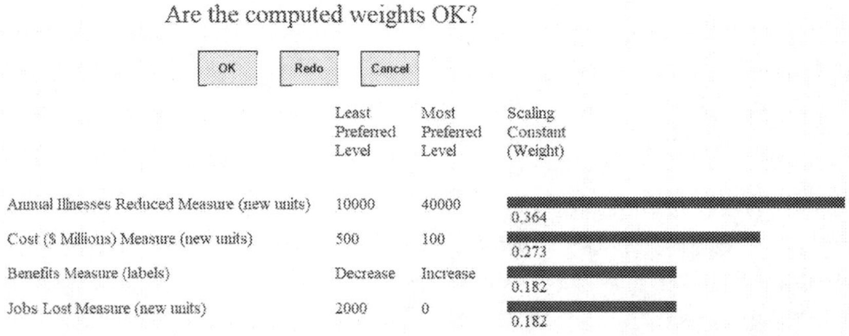

Are the computed weights OK?
OK
Redo
Cancel
Least Preferred Level
Most Preferred Level
Scaling Constant (Weight)
Annual Illnesses Reduced Measure (new units)
10000
40000
0.364
Cost ($ Millions) Measure (new units)
500
100
0.273
Benefits Measure (labels)
Decrease
Increase
0.182
Jobs Lost Measure (new units)
2000
0
0.182

*Figure 3.9* Assigning subjective weights to MCDA decision criteria.

A simple example based on the comparison in Table 3.2 is illustrated in the following discussion using Logical Decisions.* The process begins with a simple model as shown in Figure 3.8. At the top is the decision objective. In the middle are the four criteria that will be used to make the decision, and alternative solutions are shown on the bottom.

Someone must specify the relative importance of the four criteria in the decision-making process. In the hypothetical example shown in Figure 3.9, assume that the weights shown reflect the decision makers' preferences. Illnesses reduced received 100 points, cost got 75 points, and the remaining criteria got 50 points each. When normalized over the [0,1] interval, the weights are as shown.

Measurements for each alternative's contribution to each criterion are also entered. These are simply the data from the comparison in Table 3.2. The MCDA process can accommodate estimates of the uncertainty in these values, although they are not used in this example. The weights assigned

* Trademark product of Logical Decisions.

Table 3.3 Consolidated SMART rating for
each of three risk management options

| Risk management option | Option score |
| --- | --- |
| RMO 1 | 0.481 |
| RMO 2 | 0.545 |
| RMO 3 | 0.500 |

by the risk manager and criteria values developed by the assessors are combined using the Simple Multi-Attribute Rating Technique (SMART) to produce scores for the three RMOs, as shown in Table 3.3.

RMO 2 is the "best" RMO based on chosen criteria, the available data and their relative weights. Figure 3.10 illustrates the trade-offs visually. RMO 2 makes the most positive contribution to two of the criteria. It is the worst on cost. MCDA does not produce answers or decisions. It produces information that can be helpful in identifying strengths and weaknesses of alternatives in light of the social values expressed in the analysis. It can be a valuable addition to a comparison process.

## 3.5.4  Making a decision

Choosing the best risk management option is the risk manager's next decision. This should be done only after taking the remaining instrumental uncertainties attending each risk management option into account. Chapter 7 presents practical methods for making decisions under uncertainty.

If the uncertainty, for any reason, is significant enough to affect the nature of the answers to the risk manager's questions, to affect the choice of a course of action, or to affect the outcome of a decision, risk managers should carefully address that circumstance. That might be done through additional research, another iteration of the risk assessment, decisions

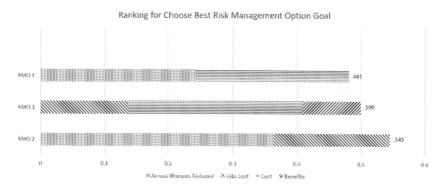

*Figure 3.10* Contribution of options to decision criteria.

phased to take advantage of the gradual resolution of key uncertainties, an adaptive management approach, or simply informed awareness of the uncertainty and its potential impacts.

The risk manager's role in the evaluation and comparison tasks is likely to be limited to deliberation. Risk assessors and others will do the relevant analysis. Making a decision based on the work done in these steps will usually be the risk manager's responsibility. In some decision contexts, the ultimate decision makers may be elected leaders or other personnel removed from or above the risk management process. Even in these instances, however, it is usual for risk managers to make a recommendation based on their experience and intimate knowledge of the problem.

## ADAPTIVE MANAGEMENT

Adaptive management is a risk management strategy that is useful when significant uncertainties can be expressed as testable risk hypotheses. Although there are many definitions, it usually consists of a series of steps that include the following:

- Identify known uncertainties at the time a decision is made.
- Include experiments that can be used to test hypotheses about the known uncertainties among the design features in the RMO.
- Measure and monitor the results of the experiments to test the identified hypotheses.
- Modify predictive models based on what is learned.
- Use the revised models to identify adjustments to the RMO actions over time to increase the likelihood that management objectives will be attained.

Adaptive management means that actions are taken to both learn about and at the same time manage the risks of interest. *Adaptive Management: The U.S. Department of the Interior Technical Guide* is an excellent resource available online (USDOI, 2009).

Risk management as described in this chapter is an iterative screening process based on scientific and other criteria. Making a decision, specifically, selecting a recommended RMO, is the final screening activity for a given risk management activity. It is in the risk control activities that the risk manager's job shifts from the normative role of describing the world as it ought to be to taking action, which is the policy dimension of the risk manager's job.

It is not unusual for some organizations to rely on default decision rules. For example, some businesses will choose the option with the minimum payback period. Doing nothing is sometimes the default action for an organization, especially one affected by the National Environmental Policy Act (NEPA). It is a safeguard that attempts to ensure that any action taken is preferable to taking no action at all.

The manner in which decisions are made cannot be fairly generalized; they will vary from organization to organization, and even within an organization they may vary from situation to situation. Good decisions are strategic; they meet objectives, avoid constraints, solve problems, and attain opportunities. Selecting an RMO is, to the extent that the RMO establishes a residual risk level, equivalent to choosing a TLR. Alternatively, there may be instances where a TLR is determined first and then RMOs are formulated to attain that specific level of risk. The same decision process described may be used for this task. No matter which way it is handled, the process and the decision itself should be carefully documented.

## 3.5.5  Identifying decision outcomes

One of the things that distinguishes risk management from other management approaches and decision-making methodologies is its focus on uncertainty. When decisions are made with less than perfect information, it is important to ask, "Is the decision working?" The answer to this question may not be evident in the near term when uncertainty is great, probabilities of occurrence are small, or time frames are long. On the other hand, we may learn quickly if our solution is working or not.

### DECISION MAKING FOR OPPORTUNITY RISKS

The concepts of acceptable and tolerable risk differ between pure and opportunity risks. When we consider these terms from the perspective of an opportunity risk, an acceptable risk is one with a negligible probability of a negative outcome or with positive consequences so large that it offsets the chance of a negative outcome. Alternatively, the negative consequences may be so slight that individuals or groups in society are willing to take or be subjected to the risk. Investing in a project that has zero chance of negative net environmental benefits might be an acceptable risk.

A tolerable opportunity risk is one that is not acceptable. Risk taking is essentially different from risk avoiding. Risk taking decisions are conscious decisions to expose oneself to a risk that could have otherwise been avoided. Consequently, managing uncertainty prior to decision making or during evolutionary decision making is a significant risk management strategy for opportunity risks.

To deal effectively with uncertainty at this level of the process, the risk manager needs to identify one or more desired outcomes of the risk management option so we can verify that the solution is working. These outcomes may relate back to the risk management objectives. We want to be able to measure the impact of our risk decision(s) on public health, the company's bottom line, ecosystems, economic activity, or other appropriate outcomes. To do this we need outcomes that are measurable in principle. In some cases, the outcome may never, in fact, be measured, but if there is any question about the effectiveness of the RMO, it could be measured. There is no effective way to discern RMOs that work from those that do not without a performance measure.

## WHO OWNS THE RISK?

Although we have spoken of risk managers as if they are all members of the same organization, that is rarely the case for decision making in the public sector. The success of an RMO may depend on many different people managing their piece of the risk.

A flood risk management (FRM) decision, for example, may require approval by and funding from Congress and the president. The U.S. Army Corps of Engineers must diligently construct all FRM structures approved by Congress. The county government may be expected to manage land use in flood hazard zones as part of the plan. State government may be responsible for operating and maintaining the FRM structures and individual residents of the flood plain may be expected to obtain flood insurance and obey evacuation orders.

A food safety risk analysis decision may involve producers, processors, wholesalers, retailers, and even consumers in the management of a risk.

Once a plan has been selected, the number of risk managers may increase markedly. They, of course, will not all have the full range of responsibilities described in this chapter but they need to understand the responsibilities they have.

### 3.5.6   Implementing the decision

Implementing an RMO means acting on the decision that was made. It requires risk managers to identify and mobilize resources necessary to actualize the RMO. Implementing a decision will very often expand the definition of who is a risk manager.

Implementation may require the cooperation of many people outside the relatively small circle of people who have worked on a risk management issue. The details of the RMO must often be implemented by a great many people. A plan to reduce traffic accidents may involve highway engineers, automobile manufacturers, drivers, and others. Reducing the number of illnesses from *Salmonella enteritidis* in shell eggs will involve farmers, food processors, transportation companies, retailers, and consumers. Many parties can own a piece of the responsibility for implementing risk management options. The specific manner of implementation will, of course, vary markedly with the nature of the risk problem and its solution.

What can we do to ensure that the various risk managers will cooperate and implement the chosen risk management strategy? This commitment is best achieved throughout the risk management process. Best practice calls for an explicit public involvement plan as part of the risk communication process for gaining commitment to the RMO. Stakeholders and the public can be expected to have an interest in the risk management decision. At a minimum, they need to know what the decision is, how it will affect them, and what their implementation responsibilities are. Most stakeholders will want to know how the decision was made and especially how trade-offs of interest to them were resolved. Risk managers must see that this communication takes place in a timely and effective manner.

## 3.6   Risk monitoring

Good RMOs can fail through faulty implementation or unravel because of false assumptions. The most brilliant strategy can be undermined if communication breaks down. Risk analysis is an evidence-based process. What is the evidence our RMO is working? If we were charged in a court room with successfully managing the risk, would there be enough evidence to convict us?

How do we know our solution works? Hubbard (2009) suggests that if we cannot answer this question, the most important thing a risk manager can do is find a way to answer it and then adopt an RMO that does work if the one currently in place does not. Figure 3.11 shows the steps comprising the last risk management task: monitoring, evaluating, and iterating.

### 3.6.1   Monitoring

It is important to provide feedback to the organization and its stakeholders on how well they are achieving their objectives. Risk managers are responsible for monitoring the outcomes of their decisions to see if they are working. There are actually three distinct things that may be

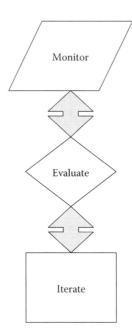

**Figure 3.11** Risk monitoring steps.

monitored in any given situation. These are decision information, decision implementation, and decision outcomes.

Some risk management decisions may not yield immediately observable outcomes. Actions taken now to change conditions in the distant future are not observable, for example, measures taken to ameliorate effects of future sea level change. Some risk problems are so uncertain that the risks themselves may be considered speculative. It is difficult to observe the reduction of risks of rare events. In these kinds of situations, it may be important to monitor information to see if data gaps are being filled. Were the underlying assumptions of the risk assessment valid? Is the risk assessment consistent with the external data? If not, are the inconsistencies known and justified? As uncertainty is reduced, a new iteration of all or part of the risk management process may be warranted. A new risk assessment, for example, may lead to better solutions in those instances where it is not yet possible to observe the effects of the RMO.

Monitoring actual implementation of the RMO is likely to be important in the near term once an organization decides to implement a specific measure. Are people doing what they are supposed to be doing? Audits can answer these questions for processes under the direct control of an organization, but when implementation requires large groups of stakeholders or the public to take or avoid certain activities, other methods of monitoring will be required. If everyone is doing what they need to do to get the RMO to work, then it is time to start monitoring outcomes.

A good risk management process will identify the outcomes to monitor in order to judge the success of an RMO. Monitoring means to watch, keep track of, or check for a special purpose. In this instance, that purpose is to determine if the desired risk reductions and other outcomes of an RMO are being achieved. In other words, "Are we meeting our risk management objectives?"

Decision makers do not always ask, "What measurable effect has our risk management option had?" The monitoring part of the risk management activity requires the risk manager to do that and to consider:

- What will we measure?
- How often will we measure?
- For how long will measurements be taken?
- Who will measure?
- What will they do with the measurements?
- Who will decide if the results are good, bad, or indifferent?
- How much will measurement cost?
- Who will pay?

It may not be necessary to begin to make these measurements immediately, but the desired outcomes (see Section 3.5.5) need to be identified before the RMO is implemented. Risk managers need to articulate for themselves and others what success looks like and how it will or could be measured. All of this should be tied directly to the risk management objectives so all can see how well they are being achieved and to allow for corrective action if necessary.

### 3.6.2 Evaluation and iteration

Once the monitoring information is gathered, it must be evaluated. This process should compare results to the original objectives to decide whether the RMO is successful. This means looking at the monitored outcomes data and judging them as satisfactory or not. One way to do this is to compare them with risk management expectations based on the risk assessment and other data. Are the desired risk reductions being achieved? Have you attained the potential benefits from your opportunities? An alternative evaluation can mean contrasting your results with what you believe is possible from other actions. Are these the best possible results? This evaluation is part of the risk manager's postimplementation responsibility.

If the evaluation step produces unsatisfactory results, the risk management decision should be modified. That modification most often will take the form of a new iteration of some or all of the risk management process. It could mean beginning again from the problem identification task, or revising and updating the risk assessment, or formulating new RMOs, or modifying the decision or its implementation strategy. The public and stakeholders should be kept informed of any and all postimplementation findings and changes in the risk management option.

Hubbard (2009) discusses four potential objective evaluations of risk management. The first is statistical inference based on a large sample. This can be a difficult way to establish the effectiveness of an option. For example, if the RMO is intended to reduce the risk of rare events, it could take a very long time indeed to compile a sample sufficient for drawing conclusions. The ability to perform risk management experiments is even more rare. Comparing results of experiments to establish the best measures is virtually unheard of in most risk management arenas. Opportunities to evaluate through statistical inference are limited by data.

Second, one can seek direct evidence of cause-and-effect relationships between our RMOs and lower risk. This approach is reasonably common in certain applications. For example, we have repeated evidence of public works projects producing the desired effects as well as of safety devices functioning as designed. Each time airport security catches a hazard at check-in, we have evidence. When a seat belt restrains a passenger, there is a clear cause-and-effect relationship.

A third method is component testing of risk management options. This method looks at the gears of risk management rather than at the entire machine. Sometimes it is possible to examine how components of the RMO have fared under controlled experiments or prior experience even if we cannot evaluate the RMO as a whole. Thus, if a pasteurization step in a food process achieves the desired log reduction in pathogens, we can have some confidence in the RMO that includes such a step.

A check of completeness is Hubbard's fourth suggestion. This technique does not measure the validity of a particular risk management method. Instead, it tries to address the question of whether the RMO is addressing a reasonably complete list of risks or risk components. You cannot manage a risk that no one has identified. Hubbard counsels risk managers to consider any list of considered risks to be incomplete.

To better ensure completeness, four perspectives should be considered: internal completeness, external completeness, historical completeness, and combinatorial completeness. Internal completeness requires the entire organization to be involved in risk identification. External completeness involves all stakeholders in identifying risks. Historical completeness considers more than recent history. It goes back as far as possible to consider potential situations of risk. Finally, the risk manager should consider combinations of events to help explore the unknown unknowns of risk.

## 3.7   Risk communication

Risk communication is a risk management responsibility that runs throughout the risk management model presented here. The risk manager need not conduct the risk communication but the risk manager is responsible for seeing that it gets done.

Risk managers must develop strategies for the internal and external communication required for successful risk management. Internal risk communication refers to essential risk communication that takes place within the risk analysis team, this is chiefly the communication between risk assessors and risk managers, although communication with risk communicators is, necessarily, a part of that process. The external communication process refers to communications between the risk analysis team and all those external to the team. Thus, external communications can involve members of the organization undertaking a specific risk management activity.

A transparent and open risk management process requires communication with all relevant stakeholders, and it is integral to good risk management decisions. This communication should include input and feedback opportunities for stakeholders as appropriate throughout the risk management activity.

It is important to make the communication process known to those with an interest in communicating. Communication must be timely. Risk managers, with the assistance of risk communicators and public involvement experts, must decide when and how to communicate. An open communication process shares what is being done to find answers to the important questions of risk managers and stakeholders. Providing public access to your data and models enhances both transparency and openness in a public-sector risk management process. Private-sector risk management will be much more circumspect. The nature of the risk communication task is addressed in Chapter 5.

## 3.8   Risk management models

Very few people have actually been educated or formally trained to be risk managers. There are an infinite variety of ways to approach all or some subset of the tasks described in this chapter. It is helpful to have mental models that inform people about how an organization handles the risk management task. In the world of risk management, there are a few

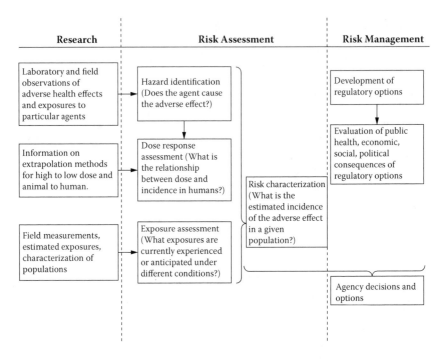

*Figure 3.12* Elements of risk assessment and risk management. (National Research Council. 1983. Committee on the Institutional Means for Assessment of Risks to Public Health. *Risk assessment in the federal government: Managing the process.* Washington, DC: National Academies Press.)

relatively generic models and many more organization- or application-specific models.

One of the earliest models of risk management, shown in Figure 3.12, comes from the "Red Book" (NRC, 1983). In the early days of risk analysis, risk assessment was the centerpiece of the risk analysis process. Figure 3.12 shows that risk assessment is supported by research. Risk management in a government regulatory context is rather crudely depicted as a matter of formulating and choosing the regulatory option to use to respond to the assessed risks.

It is not much of a stretch to suggest that in the early days of risk analysis, the general recognition of the existence of a risk initiated the conduct of a risk assessment. Risk management was more of a reaction to the risk assessment than the proactive, directive, and foundational step it is becoming today.

One of the first more evolved generic risk management models offered in the United States was developed by the Presidential/Congressional Commission on Risk Assessment and Risk Management (1997). It is shown

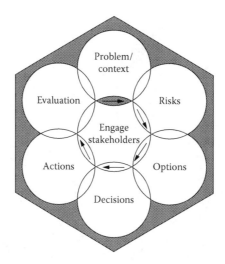

*Figure 3.13* Risk management framework of the Presidential/Congressional Commission on Risk Assessment and Risk Management.

in Figure 3.13. It begins with defining the problem and decision context and proceeds through a series of seven mostly distinct steps in an iterative fashion.

Once the problem is defined, risks are identified and assessed, RMOs are formulated, and the best option is chosen in the decisions step. Implementation occurs in a series of actions, and the success of the RMO is subsequently evaluated. This can lead to another iteration of the risk management process. At the center of the process is stakeholder involvement.

One of the more widely applied risk management models was developed by the International Organization for Standardization (ISO), ISO 31000, *Risk Management—Principles and Guidelines* (ISO, 2009). The basic model is shown in Figure 3.14. It is not specific to any industry or sector, and it can be applied to any type of risk, whatever its nature, whether it has positive or negative consequences. The model shown is quite consistent with the content of this chapter. The ISO risk management model has been updated and is revisited in Chapter 6. Be forewarned that ISO defines many terms rather differently but at its heart is consistent with the process described in this chapter.

The ISO model has five steps and two ongoing processes as well as documentation, as seen in Figure 3.14. It begins by establishing the decision context. This is followed by three steps that comprise the risk assessment process. Risks are identified and then qualitatively or quantitatively described in an analytical step (not to be confused with the overall risk

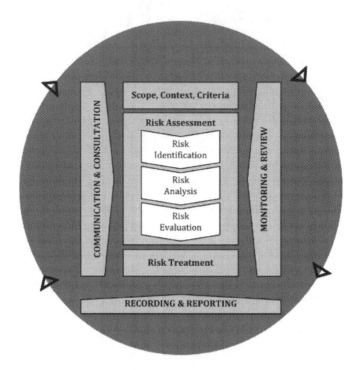

**Figure 3.14** International Organization for Standardization risk management framework.

analysis process) that produces information that enables risk evaluation. Risk treatment involves selecting one or more options for modifying risks and then implementing those options. Communication and consultation among managers and assessors as well as with external stakeholders takes place throughout the process. Monitoring and review embodies the iterative nature of this risk management process as well as the kinds of tasks discussed in the body of this chapter.

In addition to these generic models, there are infinite varieties of application/organization-specific risk management models. One such model is presented in Figure 3.15 as an example. This model is a microbiological risk management model (FAO, 2003) to be applied to food safety problems. The details of this model are less important than the greater point that there is no one right way to do risk management. There are generic models that can be adapted for specific use; the model presented in this chapter and the ISO 31000 model are good examples. In addition, there are any number of organization/industry/application-specific models. The best of all of these embody most if not all of the tasks described previously in this chapter.

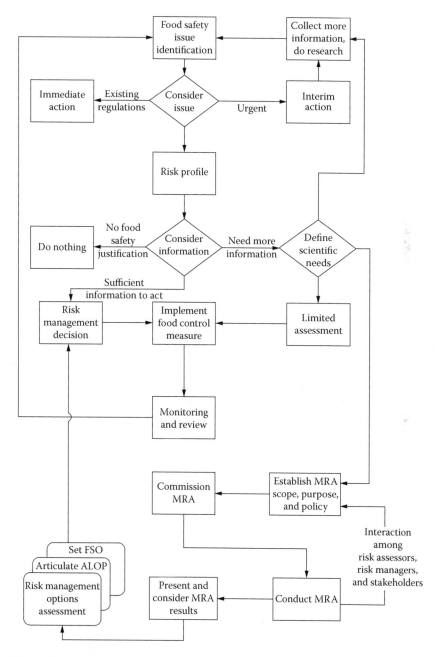

***Figure 3.15*** Microbiological risk management model. (Food and Agricultural Organization. 2003. United Nations. *Guidelines for microbiological risk management.* Orlando, FL: Codex Committee on Food Hygiene.)

What is most important for any organization that seeks to do risk analysis is to develop its own risk management model or adapt and adopt one of the existing models. Risk management is a process. People must know and use the process; that means the organization must have one!

## 3.9   Summary and look forward

To do successful risk analysis, you must have a risk management process. Then you must spend time working your process. Risk management begins and ends the risk analysis process. The risk manager's job may be described by the responsibilities they have in identifying risk, estimating risk, evaluating risk, controlling risk, and monitoring risk. You have to spend time on each of these activities to do good risk management.

Ultimately, the risk manager's job is to make effective and practical decisions under conditions of uncertainty. Establishing a process that ensures that the best available evidence is gathered, analyzed, and considered is the risk manager's responsibility. Carefully considering the instrumental uncertainties encountered in a risk management activity and seeing that their potential effects are carefully communicated to all interested parties is a primary responsibility of the risk manager.

The next chapter continues to unpack and explain the components of the risk analysis process. The practice of risk assessment is endlessly varied because of the broad and growing number of applications of the risk analysis paradigm. Risk assessment is where the initial focus of the evolving risk analysis paradigm was concentrated. In fact, there are many practitioners who would argue vociferously that risk assessment is still the heart of risk analysis. Consistent with the aim of this text, the common elements of many of these risk assessment models are identified and presented.

## References

Bernstein, P.L. 1996. *Against the Gods: The Remarkable Story of Risk*. New York: John Wiley & Sons.

Environmental Protection Agency (EPA). 1985. Office of Air Quality Planning and Standards. *Compilation of air pollution emissions factors*. Washington, DC: EPA.

Environmental Protection Agency (EPA). 1992a. Risk Assessment Forum. *Framework for ecological risk assessment*. Washington, DC: EPA.

Environmental Protection Agency (EPA). 1992b. Prepared for the Technical Workgroup, Ostrava (former Czechoslovakia), and EPA by IEC, Inc., and Sullivan Environmental Consulting. *Project Silesia: Comparative risk screening analysis*. Washington, DC: EPA.

Environmental Protection Agency (EPA). 1994. Prepared for the Technical Workgroup, Katowice, Poland, and USEPA by IEC, Inc., and Sullivan Environmental Consulting. *Project Silesia: Comparative risk screening analysis*. Washington, DC: EPA.

Environmental Protection Agency (EPA). 2010. *Thesaurus of terms used in microbial risk assessment.* https://ofmpub.epa.gov/sor_internet/registry/termreg/searchandretrieve/termsandacronyms/search.do?search=&term=RISK%20MANAGEMENT&matchCriteria=Begins&checkedAcronym=true&checkedTerm=true&hasDefinitions=false.

Food and Agricultural Organization (FAO). 2003. United Nations. *Guidelines for microbiological risk management.* Orlando, FL: Codex Committee on Food Hygiene.

Food and Drug Administration (FDA). 2003a. Center for Food Safety and Applied Nutrition. *CFSAN's risk management framework.* College Park, MD: CFSAN.

Food and Drug Administration (FDA). 2003b. *Quantitative Assessment of Relative Risk to Public Health from Foodborne Listeria monocytogenes Among Selected Categories of Ready-to-Eat Foods.* https://www.fda.gov/food/foodscienceresearch/risksafetyassessment/ucm183966.htm.

Hubbard, D.W. 2009. *The failure of risk management: Why it's broken and how to fix it.* Hoboken, NJ: John Wiley and Sons.

International Organization of Standardization (ISO). 2009. *Risk management—principles and guidelines.* Geneva, Switzerland: International Organization of Standardization.

National Research Council (NRC). 1983. Committee on the Institutional Means for Assessment of Risks to Public Health. *Risk assessment in the federal government: Managing the process.* Washington, DC: National Academies Press.

Peterson, M. 2002. What is a de minimis risk? *Risk Management* 4 (2): 47–55.

Presidential/Congressional Commission on Risk Assessment and Risk Management. 1997. *Framework for environmental health risk management final report.* Vol. 1 and 2. Washington, DC: www.riskworld.com. http://riskworld.com/nreports/1997/risk-rpt/pdf/EPAJAN.PDF.

U.S. Agency for International Development (USAID). 1990. *Ranking environmental health risks in Bangkok, Thailand.* Washington, DC: AID.

U.S. Agency for International Development (USAID). 1993a. Environmental Health Division, Office of Nutrition and Health. *Environmental health assessment: An integrated methodology for rating environmental health problems.* Washington, DC: AID.

U.S. Agency for International Development (USAID). 1993b. *Office of Health, Bureau for Research and Development.* Environmental health assessment: A case study conducted in the city of Quito and the county of Pedro Moncayo, Pichincha Province, Ecuador. WASH Field Report No. 401. Washington, DC: AID.

U.S. Agency for International Development (USAID). 1994. *Comparing environmental health risks in Cairo, Egypt.* Washington, DC: AID.

U.S. Department of the Interior (USDOI). 2009. *Adaptive management: The U.S. Department of the Interior technical guide.* Washington, DC: DOI. https://www2.usgs.gov/sdc/doc/DOI-%20Adaptive%20ManagementTechGuide.pdf.

Wingspread Conference, January, 1998. http://sehn.org/wingspread-conference-on-the-precautionary-principle/.

World Bank. 1994. *Thailand: Mitigating pollution and congestion impacts in a high-growth economy.* Washington, DC: World Bank.

Yoe, C. 2002. *Trade-off analysis planning and procedures guidebook.* IWR Report 02-R-2. Alexandria, VA: Institute for Water Resources.

*chapter four*

# Risk assessment

## 4.1 Introduction

Risk assessment pursues truth. Some risk assessments require science to discern that truth. In private sector organizations, many risk assessments simply require sound evidence to know the truth. The absolute truth is usually opaque, because of uncertainty. Good risk assessment tells the truth about what we know and what we do not know. It is the science-based component of risk analysis that provides the evidence for decision makers. It answers the risk manager's questions about the risks. It provides the objective information needed for decision making, including a characterization of the instrumental uncertainty that could influence the decision or its outcome. An assessment is done to gain an understanding of the risk(s) and to measure and describe them to the fullest extent possible. A good risk assessment meets the information needs of risk managers for decision making. It provides an objective, unbiased treatment of the available evidence in well-organized and easy to understand documentation that clearly links the evidence to its conclusions. It also describes and addresses uncertainty in intentional ways.

Risk assessment is based on orderly reasoning. It is a set of logical, systematic, evidence-based analytical activities designed to provide risk managers with the best possible identification and description of the risk(s) associated with the decision problem. Evidence can be considered to include anything that helps assessors and managers discern the truth about matters of concern to them. Risk assessment is a methodical process with specific steps that provide for a thorough and consistent approach to the assessment of risks. It meets the manager's specific decision-making needs for timing, quality, and comprehensiveness of evidence. It also provides a thorough appreciation for the uncertainties that attend those risks. Because it includes the best available scientific knowledge, it is science-based.

**SCALABLE RISK ASSESSMENT?**

In practice, you can find that there are risk assessments that warrant the complete treatment described in this chapter and there are risk assessments that require little more than the application of a specific risk assessment tool. Risk assessment can take months or years and a team of people with a very large budget or it may take one person with a risk matrix an hour or so, as well as everything between these two extremes.

This chapter describes a process that is suitable for any risk assessment effort, although it is presented as if for a substantial analytical effort. The process is, of course, perfectly scalable and its steps are as suitable for that multiyear effort as it is for the one-hour effort.

This chapter begins by considering what makes a good risk assessment. This is followed by a few definitions. Risk assessment models and techniques vary widely from one application to the next. The common elements of these have been distilled into a generic set of risk assessment activities, the description of which comprises the bulk of the chapter. Several specific risk assessment models are presented to illustrate the manner in which some communities of practice have formalized the assessment process. The chapter concludes with a brief description of the differences between qualitative and quantitative risk assessment.

## 4.2    What makes a good risk assessment?

During the 1990s, I offered a week-long course in risk assessment through the U.S. Department of Agriculture Graduate School. On Friday afternoon, I always had a panel of practitioners come in and speak about what makes a good risk assessment. I sat in the back of the room and took notes. Those notes are summarized below in 14 aspects of a good risk assessment process (see text box).

A good risk assessment gets the questions right, then answers them carefully. Good risk assessment begins with the questions risk managers would like to have answered in order to manage the risk. These are to be answered by the risk assessment. In best practice, risk assessors will understand the entire decision context and help ensure that risk managers get the questions right. Good risk assessment answers the questions clearly and concisely.

Risk assessment is usually a team sport. Evidence-based analysis requires subject-matter experts. It is unusual, but certainly not unheard of, for a single person to be able to complete a risk assessment. As risk analysis grows in acceptance, the number of routine risk assessment applications likewise increases. The more complex and unique risk assessments are never completed by a single person. Good teams are at least multidisciplinary. Better teams are interdisciplinary. The best teams are transdisciplinary.

## WHAT MAKES A GOOD RISK ASSESSMENT?

Here are the 14 aspects of a good risk assessment described in this section.

| | |
|---|---|
| Questions | Sensitivity |
| Team | Relevant Risks |
| Magnitude of Effort | Qualities |
| Point of View | Results |
| Science/Assumption | Evaluation |
| Data | Education |
| Uncertainty | Documentation |

Multidisciplinary teams ensure that the needed expertise is available. Experts on these teams tend to function as experts in isolation of one another's disciplines. The knowledge tends to be integrated by one or a few individuals. This stands in contrast to the interdisciplinary team, where all the experts integrate their knowledge with that of others. Engineers understand something about economics, and economists understand a little engineering. Biologists know a little about what the statistician is doing, and the statistician knows some biology. The team itself is integrating the knowledge of its member experts. An interdisciplinary team works more efficiently and effectively than a multidisciplinary team. A transdisciplinary team dissolves the boundaries among disciplines and moves beyond integration to assimilation of perspectives. In the process, they are often able to construct knowledge and understanding that transcends the individual disciplines. Transdisciplinary teams are preferred, but they are still rare.

The best teams spend time together working on substantive issues of common interest. Good assessment teams are collaborative and effective. Roles and responsibilities are well defined and conscientiously executed. The team answers the risk manager's questions.

The magnitude of a good assessment effort is commensurate with the resources available and in proportion to the seriousness of the problem. The effort should reflect the level of risk. Risk analysis in general and risk assessment in particular are perfectly scalable processes. A good risk assessment process can be completed in an hour if that is all the time you have or in a couple of years if that is what is warranted—the attendant uncertainty will vary markedly between these situations. The assessment process does not have to take months or years and millions of dollars, but there may be a lot of uncertainty in a quick one.

The process itself is often as valuable as the result. The process provides a basis for trust as well as for information. The process aids the understanding of the problem and its solutions. The process has to be sufficient to allow for answers to the questions posed by risk managers.

A good risk assessment has no point of view. It yields the same answers to the same questions regardless of who finances or sponsors the assessment. Although a question from the risk managers may, appropriately, reflect a point of view, the answer never should. It is not the assessor's job to protect the children, to make a product look profitable, to punish or reward anyone. It is to provide objective evidence-based answers to the questions they have been asked.

On a related note, assessors should not pursue their own curiosity in a risk assessment. Nor should they ever pursue a desired answer to any question. An assessment should never be designed to provide analysis to support a predetermined answer. If risk managers know what they want to do, a risk assessment is not necessary. Not every decision requires a risk assessment. Those that do, begin with the questions that are objectively answered.

Good risk assessment separates what we know from what we do not know, and it focuses special attention on what we do not know. Risk assessment is not pure science. The existence of uncertainty often prevents it from being so, but good risk assessment gets the right science into the assessment and then it gets that science right. Science provides the basis for answering the risk manager's questions. Honesty about uncertainty provides the confidence bounds on those answers.

Good science, good data, good models, and the best available evidence are integral to good risk assessment. Assessors need to tie their analysis to the evidence and to take care to ensure the validity of the data they use. It is both useful and important to know that not all data are quantitative. Likewise, data are not information. Skilled assessors are needed to extract the information value from data in ways that are useful and meaningful to risk managers. The answers to the risk manager's questions stand or fall on the quality of the information used to answer the questions.

It is the way that risk analysis handles the things we do not know that makes it such a useful and distinctive decision-making paradigm. In a good risk assessment, all assumptions are clearly identified for the benefit of other members of the assessment team, risk managers, and anyone else who will read or rely upon the results of the risk assessment. Risk assessors should not rely on their own default assumptions. If any default assumptions are to be used, they should be identified in the organization's risk assessment policy, prepared by risk managers.

There is uncertainty in every decision context. Risk assessors must recognize the uncertainty that exists. Moreover, they need to identify the instrumental uncertainties that influence the answers to questions, describe their significance for decision making and decision outcomes, and then address these uncertainties appropriately throughout the risk assessment. There has always been uncertainty in decision making. In the past, including the recent past, it has been commonplace to overlook or ignore the existence of uncertainty, often to the regret of those affected by decisions made this way. Admitting the things that one does not know when making a decision has often been perceived as a weakness. We like confident and bold decision makers. But we also like decisions that produce good outcomes, and the two are not always compatible. Uncertainty analysis is a strength of good risk assessment, not a weakness. Good risk assessment addresses knowledge uncertainty and natural variability in the risk assessment inputs. Good risk management addresses the variation, that is, the remaining uncertainty, in risk assessment outputs.

Sensitivity analysis should be a part of every risk assessment, qualitative or quantitative. Testing the sensitivity of assessment results, including the answers to the risk manager's questions, to changes in the assumptions assessors made to deal with the uncertainties they encountered is a minimum requirement for every assessment. Explaining how this uncertainty could affect decision making or the outcomes of decisions is the endgame for sensitivity analysis. The scenarios used to describe the risks we assess must reflect reality. That means they should be based on good science and field experience. Risk assessors need to understand how answers to the risk manager's questions might change if realizations of risk assessment inputs were to change due to their uncertainty.

## ASSUMPTIONS

No risk assessment can be completed unless the evidence is supplemented with assumptions. Explicit assumptions are those that assessors consciously make. In principle, they can be readily documented.

Implicit assumptions are those that escape the conscious awareness of the assessors. They may be based on the culture of the organization, the beliefs of the assessors, the basic assumptions, principles, and theories of the different disciplines employed, and so on. They are rarely documented. An independent review of a risk assessment by a multidisciplinary review panel can often be effective in picking up implicit assumptions, because the implicit assumptions of one discipline or person often conflict with those of another discipline or person and, thus, stand out.

All significant assumptions, whether explicit or implicit, need to be conveyed to the risk managers and other users of the assessment.

The risk assessment should address all the relevant risks. Risk is everywhere. Zero risk is not an option for any of us. Risk assessment is different from safety analysis, although safety analysis is an integral part of some risk assessments. To distinguish risk assessment from safety analysis, we need to consider risk broadly and focus on the risks of interest. These may include:

- Existing risk
- Future risk
- Historical risk
- Risk reduction
- New risk
- Residual risk
- Transferred risk
- Transformed risk

It will not always be necessary to consider each of these kinds of risk but it is rarely adequate to consider only one of these kinds of risk. Good risk assessment considers both the explicit and implicit risks relevant to the questions posed by risk managers.

Good risk assessments share some qualities in common. First, they are unbiased and objective. They tell the truth about what is known and not known about the risks. They are as transparent and as simple as possible but no simpler. Practicality, logic, comprehensiveness, conciseness, clarity, and consistency are additional qualities desired in a risk assessment. Of course, a risk assessment must be relevant. To be relevant, it must answer the questions risk managers have asked.

Risk assessments may produce more estimates and insights than scientific facts. The assessment results provide information to risk managers; they do not always produce the truth and they never produce decisions. Risk managers make decisions. The best assessments evaluate their own assumptions and judgments and convey that information to risk managers and other interested parties often in the form of confidence or uncertainty ratings. A good process makes the assessment open to evaluation. It is often wise to submit a controversial or important risk assessment to an independent evaluation or peer review.

Good risk assessments can have educational value. They often identify the limits of our knowledge and in so doing guide future research. They can help direct resources to narrowing information gaps. They help us learn about the problems, our objectives, and the right questions to ask. Completed risk assessments may be conducive to learning about similar or related risks.

There may be more than one audience for the risk assessment. Each audience is likely to have different information needs and they may each require separate documentation. This makes documentation an important part of the risk assessment process. Effective documentation tells a good story well. It is explained in simple terms and is readable by the intended audience. A good document is clear and spells important details out in terms the audience can understand. Scientific details are often most appropriately presented in technical appendices. Most important, a good risk assessment lays out the answers to the risk manager's questions clearly, well, and simply.

## *4.3   Risk assessment defined*

At its simplest, risk assessment is estimating the risks associated with different hazards, opportunities for gain, or risk management options. Many definitions of risk assessment simply identify the steps that comprise the assessment process for that application. No one definition is going to meet the needs of the many and disparate uses of risk assessment. Nonetheless, it can be informative to consider a few formal definitions.

---

**RISK ASSESSMENT LANGUAGE IS ALSO MESSY**

The World Organization for Animal Health (OIE) defines risk assessment as follows:

The evaluation of the likelihood and the biological and economic consequences of entry, establishment, or spread of a pathogenic agent within the territory of an importing country.

It has four steps:

1. Release assessment
2. Exposure assessment
3. Consequence assessment
4. Risk estimation

The International Plant Protection Convention of the United Nations defines risk assessment as "Determination of whether a pest is a quarantine pest and evaluation of its introduction potential."

ISO Guide 73:2009, definition 3.4.1 defines risk assessment as the overall process of risk identification, risk analysis, and risk evaluation.

There are no generally agreed upon definitions for risk assessment. Fortunately, the ability to develop useful and serviceable definitions for specific organizations and applications has rendered the need for a single generic definition moot. Feel free to adopt, adapt, or invent your own definition if it helps you describe the risk(s) of interest to you.

The seminal definition may be found in *Risk Assessment in the Federal Government: Managing the Process* (NRC, 1983, p. 19). This book, known widely as the "Red Book," for its cover, represents the first formal attempt to provide a description of the risk assessment process. The risks of primary interest at the time were chemical risks found in the human environment. Risk assessment was initially defined as follows: "Risk assessment can be divided into four major steps: hazard identification, dose-response assessment, exposure assessment, and risk characterization."

The steps are described by the National Research Council (NRC) as follows:

- *Hazard identification*: the determination of whether a particular chemical is or is not causally linked to particular health effects
- *Dose-response assessment*: the determination of the relation between the magnitude of exposure and the probability of occurrence of the health effects in question
- *Exposure assessment*: the determination of the extent of human exposure before or after application of regulatory controls
- *Risk characterization*: the description of the nature and often the magnitude of human risk, including attendant uncertainty.

## RISK ASSESSMENT

When asked to name the riskiest things they do, most people will quickly identify driving. A simple risk assessment process can be demonstrated by asking the four questions used to define risk assessment in Chapter 1.

What can go wrong? One could have an accident.

What are the consequences? Property damage, injury, fatalities, or perhaps only delay and annoyance could result from an accident.

How can it happen? The driver could be impaired, road or weather conditions could be hazardous, the car could be poorly maintained.

How likely is it? Perhaps knowing yourself you might say, not very likely.

That is a risk assessment process. Is it good enough to run an insurance company or to design highways? Of course not! However, it is perfectly adequate to demonstrate the idea of a scalable and systematic process. Given more time, resources, and importance all of the answers could be expanded and quantified.

### STEM

Cox (2002) says a risk can be defined by answering the following four questions:

- What is the **source** of the risk?
- What or who is the **target** that is at risk?
- What is the adverse **effect** of concern that the source may cause in exposed targets?
- By what causal **mechanism** does the source increase the probability of the effect in exposed targets?

These definitions have been and continue to be the focal point for many definitions of risk assessment. The *Codex Alimentarius*, for example, defined risk assessment for food safety purposes in 2004 as follows: "Risk Assessment: A scientifically based process consisting of the following steps: (i) hazard identification, (ii) hazard characterization, (iii) exposure assessment, and (iv) risk characterization" (FAO/WHO, 2004, p. 45). The roots of the original definition are clearly evident in this one, which has simply broadened the notion of using a dose-response assessment to characterize the consequences of exposure to a hazard.

The NRC definition as broadened by the *Codex* has a lot of appeal for risk assessors. It begins by identifying the hazard, which is the thing or activity that can cause harm. The hazard characterization step describes the nature of that harm and the conditions required to cause it. The exposure assessment describes the manner in which people or other assets of value can become exposed to the hazard under conditions that will cause harm. The last step, risk characterization, pulls together the information in the three preceding steps to describe the probability that the risk will occur as well as the severity of its consequences.

The Presidential/Congressional Commission on Risk Assessment and Risk Management (1997a, 1997b) defined risk assessment more generally. It said that risk assessment is the systematic, scientific characterization of potential adverse effects of human or ecological exposures to hazardous agents or activities. It is performed by considering the types of hazards, the extent of exposure to the hazards, and information about the relationship between exposures and responses, including variation in susceptibility. Adverse effects or responses could result from exposures to chemicals, microorganisms, radiation, or natural events. This definition did not catch on with federal agencies in the United States because it did not meet the widely varying needs of the agencies using risk assessment.

ISO 31000 *Risk Management—Principles and Guidelines* (ISO, 2009) defines risk assessment as the overall process of risk identification, risk analysis, and risk evaluation. Beware the messy language of risk! Risk identification is the process of finding, recognizing, and describing risks. Risk analysis is a process to comprehend the nature of risk and to determine the level of risk. It is equivalent to risk assessment as described in this chapter. Risk evaluation is the process of comparing the results of risk analysis with risk criteria to determine whether the risk and/or its magnitude is acceptable or tolerable. The Society for Risk Analysis defines risk assessment as a systematic process to comprehend the nature of risk, express and evaluate risk, with the available knowledge.

For the general purposes of this book, risk assessment is defined as a systematic evidence-based process for describing (qualitatively or quantitatively) the nature, likelihood, and magnitude of risk associated with some substance, situation, action, or event that includes consideration of relevant uncertainties. The generic assessment steps adopted for this book are shown in Figure 4.1.

Risk assessment is a continuously evolving process with a stable core that takes many forms, as evidenced by the previous definitions and the models that follow in this chapter. The core of risk assessment may best be described by the four informal questions introduced in Chapter 1:

- What can go wrong?
- What are the consequences?
- How can it happen?
- How likely is it to happen?

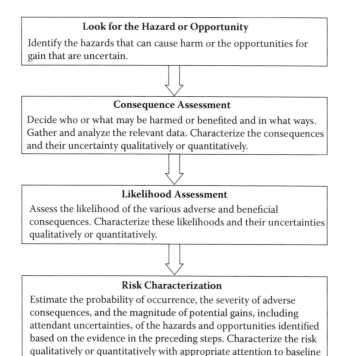

**Look for the Hazard or Opportunity**
Identify the hazards that can cause harm or the opportunities for gain that are uncertain.

**Consequence Assessment**
Decide who or what may be harmed or benefited and in what ways. Gather and analyze the relevant data. Characterize the consequences and their uncertainty qualitatively or quantitatively.

**Likelihood Assessment**
Assess the likelihood of the various adverse and beneficial consequences. Characterize these likelihoods and their uncertainties qualitatively or quantitatively.

**Risk Characterization**
Estimate the probability of occurrence, the severity of adverse consequences, and the magnitude of potential gains, including attendant uncertainties, of the hazards and opportunities identified based on the evidence in the preceding steps. Characterize the risk qualitatively or quantitatively with appropriate attention to baseline and residual risks, risk reductions, transformations, and transfers.

*Figure 4.1* Four generic risk assessment components.

## 4.4   Risk assessment activities

The great variety of risk assessment models, methods, and applications makes it difficult to speak about risk assessment in a way with which all will agree. I describe the risk assessment component of risk analysis by breaking it down into eight generic risk assessment tasks that appear to varying extents in one form or another in all best-practice risk assessment. They are shown in Figure 4.2 and are addressed in the sections that follow.

The tasks, although presented in a linear fashion, are often accomplished in an iterative fashion. Some tasks may be initiated simultaneously, for example, the consequence and likelihood assessments may be done concurrently. It is less important that the tasks be accomplished in a rigid fashion than that all of the tasks get done at least once.

### 4.4.1   Understand the questions

In case you had not picked up on the importance of questions from earlier in the chapter, risk assessors need to understand what information they

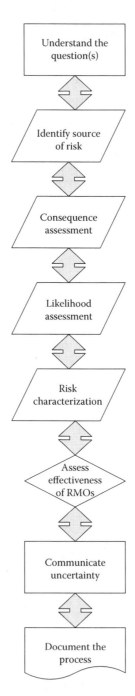

*Figure 4.2* Eight risk assessment tasks.

are being asked to provide back to risk managers. Assessors are often involved in helping risk managers to identify the questions that need to be answered for risk managers to achieve their risk management objectives and solve their problems. Questions are just one common way of eliciting information that is needed for decision making. Questions need not literally be questions. Information needs can be expressed in any number of ways. Whether assessors are involved or not, obtaining a preliminary set of the questions to be answered by the risk assessment is the essential starting point for any risk assessment.

Assessors should review the questions with the managers to make sure they have a common understanding of the meaning of the questions and the information required to answer them. If the assessors know it is going to be impossible to answer some of the questions, they need to tell the risk managers this. A revised set of questions needs to be negotiated and approved by the managers. If important questions are missing, assessors should argue for their inclusion.

## SOME REAL QUESTIONS

What is known about the dose-response relationship between consumption of *Vibrio parahaemolyticus* and illnesses?

What is the frequency and extent of pathogenic strains of *Vibrio parahaemolyticus* in shellfish waters and in oysters?

What environmental parameters (e.g., water temperature, salinity) can be used to predict the presence of *Vibrio parahaemolyticus* in oysters?

How do levels of *Vibrio parahaemolyticus* in oysters at harvest compare to levels at consumption?

What is the role of post-harvest handling on the level of *Vibrio parahaemolyticus* in oysters?

What reductions in risk can be anticipated with different potential intervention strategies?

**Source: Quantitative Risk Assessment on the Public Health Impact of Pathogenic *Vibrio parahaemolyticus* in Raw Oysters (FDA, 2005)**

Some organizations face recurring situations or they handle a specific kind of risky situation as a matter of routine. In these instances, the specific questions to be answered may be well known and long established. For example, the Animal Plant Health Inspection Service (APHIS) of the U.S. Department of Agriculture routinely processes requests from countries that would like to export their plants and plant products to the United States. APHIS has developed a standardized risk assessment process that relies on a well-defined set of questions that is used for all such routine requests.

The U.S. Army Corps of Engineers routinely addresses flood problems across the country. No two of them are alike, but flood risk management investigations are similar enough that many of the information needs have become standardized. Estimating what the expected annual flood damages are with and without risk management measures in place are universal questions that have been standardized in guidance documents and practice.

The food-additive safety assessment process has a well-established procedure for assessing health risks of chemicals added to food. It begins by undertaking toxicity studies of the substance. These studies are used to determine the "No Observed Adverse Effect Level" (NOAEL). A safety or uncertainty factor is used to extrapolate the NOAEL results from animals to humans. Dividing the NOAEL by the safety factor yields an Acceptable Daily Intake (ADI). This is the maximum amount the average human can consume daily for a lifetime with no adverse health effect. Simultaneous efforts to calculate the Estimated Daily Intake (EDI) of the substance are undertaken, and the two are compared via the ratio, EDI/ADI. Values greater than 1 require risk management. These data input requirements are well established.

## SELECTED SOURCES OF SCIENTIFIC INFORMATION FOR RISK ASSESSMENTS

- Published scientific studies
- Professional literature
- Specific research studies designed to fill data gaps
- Administrative data and internal documents
- Gray literature–unpublished studies and surveys carried out by academia, government, industry, and nongovernmental agencies
- National and other monitoring data
- National human health surveillance and laboratory diagnostic data
- Disease outbreak investigations
- National, published and proprietary surveys, inventories and the like
- Expert panels to elicit expert opinion where specific data sets are not available
- Risk assessments carried out by others
- International databases
- International risk assessments

Thus, the risk manager's data needs may already be well established for some risk assessments. These will usually be available in official policy, guidance, or common practice. In other unique instances, risk managers will have to carefully articulate each of their data needs. The majority of risk assessments may well fall between these two extremes. Regardless of the individual circumstances of an assessment, the risk manager's questions should be written down and understood by all. These questions guide the risk assessment.

## 4.4.2 Identify the source of the risk

Data collection and analysis begin in earnest when risk assessors seek to identify, understand, and describe the source of the harm that could occur or the gain that may be realized. The source of the risk—the hazards that can cause harm or the opportunities for gain that are uncertain—may already have been identified, as the decision context was established by the managers, with or without the assistance of the assessors, especially if a risk profile was prepared first. It is usual for assessors to participate in the preparation of a risk profile.

In many risk assessment models, this step is called "hazard identification." For Environmental Protection Agency (EPA) Superfund risks, this is the process of determining whether exposure to a chemical agent can cause an increase in the incidence of a particular adverse health effect (e.g., cancer, birth defects) and whether the adverse health effect is likely to occur in humans. For food safety concerns, it may mean identifying a pathogen-commodity pair that is of concern. For engineering projects, it may mean describing an earthquake or coastal storm risk, or it could be determining the demand on a structural component relative to its capacity. For APHIS, it may include identifying a pest of potential quarantine concern. For a pharmaceutical firm, it may be impurities or irregularities in the production of a drug. It could also mean identifying the potential gains from an investment in tourism or the gain associated with opening a new store or launching a new product line. In enterprise risk management it could be anything that threatens a firm's ability to meet its strategic objectives.

### TWO CONSEQUENCE CAVEATS

Managers and assessors need to remain vigilant against imprecise language. It is easy to ask: What is the risk associated with eating oysters contaminated with pathogenic *Vibrio parahaemolyticus*? But what are the consequences of concern to risk managers? Is it annual deaths, hospitalizations, illnesses, or exposures? Should they be segregated by age, gender, ethnicity, or other factors? Do we want estimates of the probability of death and illness? If so, should they be per exposure or annually? Or are other measures like loss of life expectancy, working days lost, and quality adjusted life years appropriate?

Managers and assessors also need to think broadly about consequences. A narrow focus on consequences can cause managers to overlook important impacts of both the risk and the RMOs. For example, if the assessment is motivated by public health consequences, it is easy to overlook important impacts on trade, industry, and consumers.

The cure for these mistakes is found in a good risk management process and those "three pieces of paper" it produces.

Identifying the source of the risk is more than simply naming a hazard or opportunity. It includes understanding the background, context, and aspects of the hazard or opportunity relevant to the problem being addressed and communicating that to others. The extent of this process will vary from situation to situation. For example, identifying a food-borne pathogen may be very straightforward for well-known microbiological hazards yet far from fully developed for emerging or new microbiological hazards. Economic opportunities may need to be supported with market studies and cost details. Technological risks need to be explained in a narrative fashion that facilitates understanding by all interested parties. In other words, assessors must gather the evidence necessary to establish the existence of a hazard or opportunity.

The risk assessor should think comprehensively about risks. This means identifying all of the decision-relevant risks. It is all too easy to focus too narrowly and too quickly on a single risk when there may in fact be more than one. It also means considering all the relevant dimensions of a risk, including not only the existing risk, but residual, new, transformed, and transferred risks. Identifying the source of a risk is primarily a qualitative analysis. Importantly, hazard/opportunity identification is the point in the risk assessment where risk assessors begin to carefully identify and separate what we know about a risk from what we do not know.

### 4.4.3   Consequence assessment

In this task, risk assessors characterize the nature of the harm caused by a hazard or the gain that is possible with an opportunity. Assessors identify who or what may be harmed or benefited and in what ways by the sources of risk identified in the previous task. This activity might be described as the cause-effect link in the risk assessment. What undesirable effects do the hazards have? What desirable effects might the opportunities offer? Risks affect human, animal, and plant life, public health, public safety, ecosystems, property, natural and cultural resources, human systems (political, legal, education, transportation, communication, and the like), business operations and bottom lines, infrastructure, economies, international trade and treaties, financial resources, and so on. Carefully identifying the consequences and linking them to the hazards and opportunities is an essential early step in any risk assessment. It also helps solidify the definition of the risk. This activity may be likened to the hazard characterization step of the *Codex* model.

The consequences of most importance should already be reflected in the "three pieces of paper" developed by risk managers before the risk assessment was initiated. In an iterative process, such as risk assessment, it is to be expected that, as uncertainty is reduced, some aspects of the assessment will become better understood. This may necessitate revising the initial assessment of relevant consequences.

Effectively managing a risk requires a broad understanding of the relevant losses, harm, consequences, and potential gains to all interested and affected parties (NRC, 1996). Consequences may be characterized qualitatively or quantitatively. No matter which type of characterization is used, it is essential to catalogue the significant uncertainties encountered in describing and linking the consequence to the source hazards and opportunities.

If the risk has not previously been carefully identified, it will be useful to identify the specific consequences of interest in the assessment before initiating the likelihood assessment. As noted earlier, it is important to answer the "likelihood of what?" question before investing much effort in assessing the likelihood. In ongoing programs with recurring types of risks, the consequences may be well defined by policy and practice that enable the assessors to conduct a simultaneous likelihood assessment.

### 4.4.3.1  Dose-response relationships

The earliest risk assessments used dose-response relationships to characterize the consequences of human health risks. Dose-response relationships, often represented as curves, remain the primary health-consequence model used to characterize the adverse human health effects of chemicals, toxins, and microbes in the environment. There is extensive literature on these dose-response relationships that includes its own journal, *Dose-Response*. A discussion of consequence assessment is not complete without a brief mention of this often-used relationship.

Consider the conceptual representation of a dose-response curve shown in Figure 4.3, adapted from Covello and Merkhofer (1993), where they described the effect of a risk agent on a large population. First, notice that the dose of the risk agent increases from left to right on the horizontal axis. The response, on the vertical axis, is not specified. In practice, this axis may be the probability of illness or of some other adverse health effect, the number of excess tumors above those observed in a control group, for example, or virtually any adverse health effect. The metrics on the vertical axis are most often developed for a representative individual of the general population, the general population itself, or any subpopulation of interest.

Five different conceptual distinctions are made in the figure to aid the general understanding of the relationship. Let us illustrate these concepts using two different responses. The first is an unspecified set of variable adverse health effects encompassing such effects as excessive salivation, elevated blood pressure, infection, organ failure, and death. The second response is lifetime probability of cancer. First, at sufficiently low doses there may be significant uncertainty about the response. "No threshold" models assume there is no absolutely safe level of exposure. However, for many risk agents there may be no effects at very low doses regardless of the duration of the exposure. At this level of exposure when the response is, say, the probability of cancer for a representative member

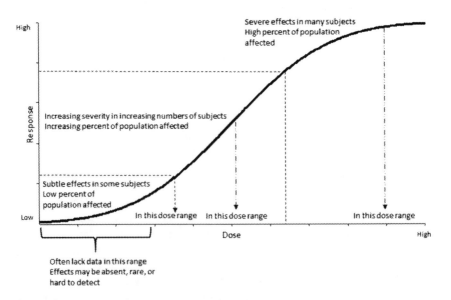

*Figure 4.3* A stylized dose-response relationship.

of the population, the shape of the curve in this range of doses may be highly uncertain.

At somewhat higher levels of exposure, subtle adverse health responses may be detected in some subjects. This might include low impact effects like excess salivation or using the probability of cancer, we would see a low but increasing probability.

As the dose increases more, we might see the beginning of some severe effects in some members of the population with a growing number of less severe effects. The cancer risk model simply has an increasing likelihood of cancer. In that fourth dose region, we would expect to see increasing numbers of severe health effects among members of the population. Both incidence and severity increase with these relatively high doses of the risk agent. If the dose increases high enough and lasts long enough, all members of the population are at risk of some adverse response. Similarly, the probability of cancer rises to higher levels. The final response range corresponding to the highest dose levels results in death or a probability of cancer approaching one.

This conceptual model is not to be taken literally. Response will not always be a continuum from no effects to death; the probability of cancer response presents one alternative. The doses themselves will vary as well. Chemical exposures, for example, may be measured in mg/kg/ body weight daily for a lifetime. Microbial doses may be measured in the number of cells or colony-forming units per some amount of food.

## 4.4.4   Likelihood assessment

Risk assessors analyze the manner in which the undesirable consequences of hazards or the desirable consequences of opportunities occur so they can characterize the likelihoods of the sequence of events that produce these outcomes. Risks cannot be directly observed or measured because they are potential outcomes that may or may not occur. Uncertain occurrence is a necessary, but not sufficient, condition for risk; an undesirable outcome is the other necessary condition. Probability is the most common language of uncertainty. Thus, qualitatively or quantitatively assessing the probability/ likelihood of the various adverse and beneficial consequences associated with the identified risks is necessary for risk assessment. This step is most analogous to the exposure assessment task of the NRC "Red Book" or *Codex* models.

Assessing the likelihoods of the consequences associated with identified risks can often be aided by developing a risk hypothesis. A risk hypothesis is a model or scenario that credibly explains how the source of the risk can lead to the consequences of concern by identifying the appropriate sequence of uncertain events that must occur for this to happen.

The likelihood assessment characterizes the chance of that sequence of events occurring. Think of this step as estimating the probability that a risk target (person or thing) will be exposed to the hazard that can cause harm. Alternatively, it is estimating the probability that an opportunity does (or does not) yield a favorable outcome.

> In the relatively loose, that is, nontechnical language of risk, probability and likelihood are used as synonyms. Some draw a nontechnical distinction that uses probability for quantitative estimates and likelihood for qualitative estimates. More rigorously, likelihood is not a probability but we yield to the use of these words as synonyms in this text.

Three simple risk hypotheses are illustrated in Figures 4.4 through 4.6. The first example in Figure 4.4 is a risk model for estimating expected annual flood damages. For the upper-right quadrant, it is assumed that property damage (consequence), measured in dollars, increases with water depth. The upper-left quadrant shows the volume of water flow (hazard) required to reach the corresponding depths of water. On the lower left, the likelihoods of the various flows being equaled or exceeded in a year are shown. These three relationships* together yield the fourth relationship (damage-frequency) in the lower-right quadrant, which when integrated provides a measure of property damages called expected annual damages. The likelihood characterization is derived from the middle two quadrants.

A second risk hypothesis is seen in Figure 4.5. This shows the presumed relationship between a human activity (logging), the stressors it creates, and the adverse effects that can result in a forest environment (EPA, 1998). A likelihood assessment would require estimating the likelihood of each of these model elements.

The risk hypothesis embodied in the FDA risk assessment on *Vibrio parahaemolyticus* in raw oysters (FDA, 2005) is shown in Figure 4.6. The likelihood characterization is more complexly woven through elements of this hypothesis.

It is essential to identify the significant uncertainties and to analyze their potential impact on the likelihoods of the risks. This may be done qualitatively or quantitatively, in concert with the level of detail in the overall risk assessment.

---

* Adapting the terminology of the NRC definition of risk assessment, the depth-damage curve is a dose-response relationship. The depth-flow and flow-frequency curves comprise an exposure assessment. The damage-frequency curve is a risk characterization.

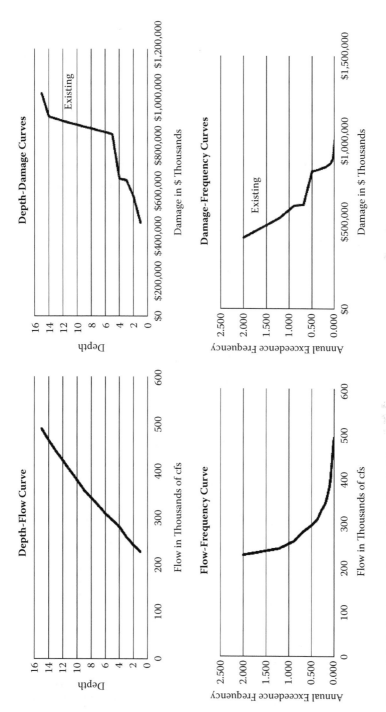

*Figure 4.4* Hydroeconomic model for flood risk.

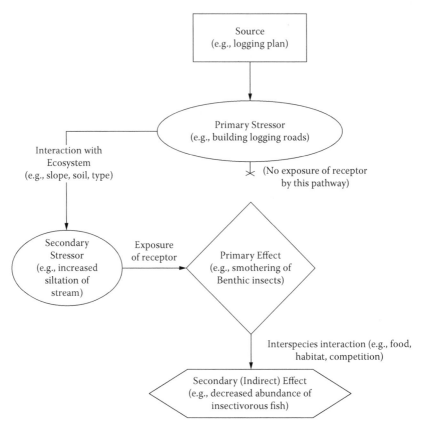

*Figure 4.5* Conceptual model for logging forest products. (From Environmental Protection Agency. 1998. *Federal Register* 63 (93): 26846–26924.)

### 4.4.4.1   *Exposure assessment*

The likelihood characterization includes the special subset of "exposure assessments" that virtually all health-related risk assessments require. An exposure assessment estimates the intensity, frequency, and duration of exposure to a risk agent. Exposure assessments identify the relevant pathways by which a human or other population is exposed to a hazard. The exposure assessment is often the most difficult part of a risk assessment, because the pathways can be both numerous and complex. They are also plagued by knowledge uncertainty and natural variability.

Exposures can be monitored directly, when direct measurement of the individual's exposure by instruments is possible. Otherwise we are restricted to measuring factors that affect exposure rather than the exposure itself. These are indirect methods of monitoring. Spatial and

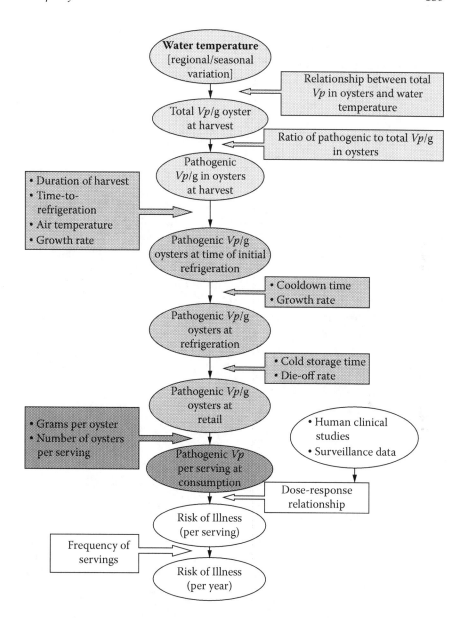

*Figure 4.6* Schematic representation of the *Vibrio parahaemolyticus* risk assessment model. (From Food and Drug Administration. 2005. *Quantitative risk assessment on the public health impact of pathogenic Vibrio parahaemolyticus in raw oysters.* College Park, MD: Center for Food Safety and Applied Nutrition. http://www.fda.gov/ Food/ScienceResearch/ResearchAreas/RiskAssessmentSafetyAssessment/ ucm050421.htm.)

temporal variations are often important considerations in exposure assessments. Models used to capture the relevant aspects of an exposure pathway can be quite complex.

A general exposure equation adapted from the EPA (Covello and Mumpower, 1985) is:

Intake =

$$\frac{\text{Concentration} \times \text{Contact rate} \times \text{Exposure frequency} \times \text{Exposure period}}{\text{Body weight}}$$

(4.1)

Here, intake is defined as mg/kg of body weight per some duration of exposure. The concentration of the risk agent (e.g., a chemical) in a medium during the exposure period is multiplied by the amount of contaminated medium contacted per unit of time or per event to get the amount of risk agent per exposure. The exposure frequency (days per year, for example) is multiplied by the exposure period (number of years) to get the duration of the exposure. The product of these two values (amount of risk agent and duration of exposure) is divided by body weight to get a dose to which one is exposed. This dose may then feed into a dose-response relationship, as discussed previously.

In the event of a microbial exposure, a general exposure equation might be:

$$\text{Intake} = \text{Concentration of pathogen per medium weight} \\ \times \text{Total weight of medium} \qquad (4.2)$$

The resulting number of cells or colony-forming units provides an estimate of the dose, which might have an associated probability of an adverse health effect if a dose-response relationship is available.

### 4.4.5   Risk characterization

Risk characterization is where many of the risk manager's questions usually get answered. Risk characterization typically includes descriptions of the probability of occurrence and the severity of adverse consequences associated with hazards, as well as the magnitude of potential gains from opportunities identified based on the evidence and analysis in all the preceding steps. Risks can be characterized qualitatively or quantitatively.

Characterizations include one or more estimates of risk and their accompanying risk descriptions. A risk estimate is an estimate of the likelihood and severity of the adverse effects or opportunities, which addresses key attending uncertainties. Quantitative estimates are numerical in nature and are usually preferred over narrative qualitative estimates. Risk estimates should include all the relevant aspects of the risk, which may encompass existing, future, historical, reduced, residual, new, transformed, and transferred risks. A risk description is a narrative explanation and depiction of a risk that bounds and defines a risk for decision-making purposes. The story that accompanies the risk estimate is what places it in a proper context for risk managers and others to understand.

There are different approaches to risk characterization. The choice of an approach depends on the needs, objectives, and questions of the risk managers. Any good risk characterization will convert the scientific evidence base into a statement of risk that answers the manager's questions. It is convenient to think of the different risk characterization approaches as running along a continuum from qualitative to quantitative. Between the two lie semi-quantitative risk characterizations, which are sometimes useful.

It is during the risk characterization that the overall importance of the various uncertainties encountered throughout the risk assessment begins to come into focus. Risk characterization should include sensitivity analysis or formal uncertainty analysis commensurate with the nature of the risk assessment.

## 4.4.6 Assess effectiveness of risk management options

In most cases, risk assessors will be asked to estimate risk reductions attributable to the risk mitigation options (RMOs) under consideration. In some situations, assessors or others may be asked for additional evaluations of the RMOs along with the evaluation of RMO efficacy. These evaluations might include economic costs and benefits, environmental impacts, social impacts, legal ramifications, and the like.

Typically, the existing level of risk is assessed, and if it is judged to be unacceptable, it will be reduced to a tolerable level if it cannot be eliminated. Often the unspoken "default" level of tolerable risk is as low as reasonably achievable. In other instances, risks are reduced to the point where the costs of further reductions clearly outweigh the benefits of additional risk reductions.

---

**EXAMPLE RISK DESCRIPTION AND RISK ESTIMATE**

The "risk per annum" is the predicted number of illnesses (gastroenteritis alone or gastroenteritis followed by septicemia) in the United States each year. As shown in the Summary Table, for each region, the highest number of predicted cases of illnesses is associated with oysters harvested in the summer and spring and the lowest in the winter and fall. Of the total annual predicted *Vibrio parahaemolyticus* illnesses, approximately 92% are attributed to oysters harvested from the Gulf Coast (Louisiana and non-Louisiana states) region in the spring, summer, and fall and from the Pacific Northwest (intertidal) region in the summer. The lower numbers of illnesses predicted for the Northeast Atlantic and Mid-Atlantic oyster harvests are attributable both to the colder water temperatures and the smaller harvest from these regions. The harvesting practice also has an impact on the illness rate. Intertidal harvesting in the Pacific Northwest poses a much greater risk than dredging in this region (192 vs. 4 illnesses per year). This is likely attributable to elevation of oyster temperatures during intertidal exposure leading to *Vibrio parahaemolyticus* growth.

**Summary Table.** Predicted mean annual number of illnesses associated with the consumption of *Vibrio parahaemolyticus* in raw oysters

| Region | Mean annual illnesses[a] | | | | |
|---|---|---|---|---|---|
| | Summer | Fall | Winter | Spring | Total |
| Gulf Coast (Louisiana) | 1406 | 132 | 7 | 505 | 2050 |
| Gulf Coast (Non-Louisiana)[b] | 299 | 51 | 3 | 193 | 546 |
| Mid-Atlantic | 7 | 4 | <1 | 4 | 15 |
| Northeast Atlantic | 14 | 2 | <1 | 3 | 19 |
| Pacific Northwest (Dredged) | 4 | <1 | <1 | <1 | 4 |
| Pacific Northwest (Intertidal)[c] | 173 | 1 | <1 | 18 | 192 |
| Total | 1903 | 190 | 10 | 723 | 2826 |

*Source: Quantitative Risk Assessment on the Public Health Impact of Pathogenic Vibrio para-*
*haemolyticus in Raw Oysters* (FDA, 2005).

[a] Mean annual illnesses refers to the predicted number of illnesses (gastroenteritis alone or gastroenteritis followed by septicemia) in the United States each year.
[b] Includes oysters harvested from Florida, Mississippi, Texas, and Alabama. The time from harvest to refrigeration in these states is typically shorter than for Louisiana.
[c] Oysters harvested using intertidal methods are typically exposed to higher temperature for longer times before refrigeration compared with dredged methods.

In some decision settings, the trade-offs among risk reduction, cost, and other criteria are more complex, and an array of RMOs may be under consideration. In these situations, it is usually desirable to use a "with" and "without" risk management option comparison, as described in the previous chapter, along with a more formal trade-off analysis.

Considering residual, new, transferred, and transformed risk at the time that risk reductions are estimated is likely to be efficient. In some instances, RMOs will be reasonably well formulated at the time that the risk assessment is initiated. In other situations, due to the iterative nature of risk analysis science, RMOs may not even be identified until well after the risk assessment has begun. In other cases, it may not even be appropriate to begin to formulate RMOs until after the risk has been initially assessed and judged to be unacceptable. For these reasons, this RMO assessment step, often considered an integral part of risk characterization in some descriptions of risk assessment, is separated out here. Uncertainties concerning the performance or efficacy of an RMO in reducing unacceptable risks to acceptable or tolerable levels should be investigated and documented so that risk managers and other interested parties may be made aware of them.

## EXAMPLE: EFFECTIVENESS OF RMOS

*Summary Table.* Predicted mean number of illnesses per annum from reduction of levels of pathogenic *Vibrio parahaemolyticus* in oysters

| Region | Predicted mean number of illnesses per annum | | | |
|---|---|---|---|---|
| | Baseline | Immediate refrigeration[a] | 2-log reduction[b] | 4.5-log reduction[c] |
| Gulf Coast (Louisiana) | 2050 | 202 | 22 | <1 |
| Gulf Coast (Non-Louisiana) | 546 | 80 | 6 | <1 |
| Mid-Atlantic | 15 | 2 | <1 | <1 |
| Northeast Atlantic | 19 | 3 | <1 | <1 |
| Pacific Northwest (Dredged) | 4 | <1 | <1 | <1 |
| Pacific Northwest (Intertidal) | 192 | 106 | 2 | <1 |
| Total | 2826 | 391 | 30 | <1 |

*Source: Quantitative Risk Assessment on the Public Health Impact of Pathogenic Vibrio parahaemolyticus in Raw Oysters* (FDA, 2005).

[a] Represents refrigeration immediately after harvest; the effectiveness of which varies both regionally and seasonally and is typically approximately 1-log reduction.
[b] Represents any process which reduces levels of *Vibrio parahaemolyticus* in oysters 2-log, for example, freezing.
[c] Represents any process which reduces levels of *Vibrio parahaemolyticus* in oysters 4.5-log, for example, mild heat treatment, irradiation, or ultrahigh hydrostatic pressure.

## 4.4.7   Communicate uncertainty

It is not enough for risk assessors to identify and investigate the significance of the instrumental uncertainties identified throughout the risk assessment. They must communicate its significance for decision making to risk managers. Methodologies for effectively conveying information about what is known with certainty and which remaining uncertainties could affect the risk characterization or the answers to the risk manager's questions need to be developed and carried out. When it comes to decision making, it is better to have a general and incomplete map, subject to revision and correction, than to have no map at all (Toffler, 1990). But those using the risk assessment map to make decisions must know its limitations.

Characterizing the significance of the instrumental uncertainties in a risk assessment is critical to informed decision making. The NRC (1994) said, "Uncertainty forces decision makers to judge how probable it is that risks will be overestimated or underestimated." This is important for risk managers to understand, as they determine the need for and appropriate choice of an RMO.

Characterizing uncertainty can also support the informed consent of those affected by risk management decisions. When people are asked to live behind a levee or near a nuclear power plant, to get a vaccination for a seasonal flu, or to board an airplane, they have a right to know the limitations of the risk management measures taken on their behalf as well as the limitations of the information on which those measures were based. Characterizing uncertainty is essential to the transparency of a risk assessment. Transparency enhances the credibility of the process, improves the defensibility of actions taken or not taken, and empowers affected individuals to make better choices for themselves in response to the risks that remain.

Uncertainty analysis also identifies important data gaps, which can be filled to improve the accuracy of the risk assessment and, hence, support improved decision making. Risk assessors should communicate their degree of confidence in the risk assessment they have done so that risk managers can take this into consideration for decision making. To do this, risk assessors should explicitly address natural variability and knowledge uncertainty and their potential impacts on the risk estimate in every risk characterization, qualitative or quantitative. All assumptions should be acknowledged and made explicit. The impacts of these assumptions on the risk characterization and subsequently the manager's use of the risk assessment in decision making are to be thoroughly discussed. Assessors should describe the strengths and limitations of the assessment along with their impacts on the overall assessment findings. Assessors should also say whether they believe the risk assessment adequately addresses the risk manager's questions.

The International Programme on Chemical Safety (IPCS, 2008) has proposed four tiers or levels of uncertainty analysis, which provide a useful way to think about this activity. These are:

- Tier 0: Default assumptions
- Tier 1: Qualitative but systematic identification and characterization of uncertainty
- Tier 2: Quantitative evaluation of uncertainty making use of bounding values, interval analysis, and sensitivity analysis
- Tier 3: Probabilistic assessment with single or multiple outcome distributions reflecting uncertainty and variability

Each of these tiers entails different responsibilities for the risk assessors. In best practice, default assumptions will rarely be used. Uncertainty can be discussed in the absence of quantitative data. It is always possible to tell decision makers what is known with certainty, what we suspect based on incomplete data, and what we assume based on inadequate or missing data. The key is to adopt a systematic approach to communicate the uncertainty qualitatively. This will help to ensure that the job is done adequately.

Quantitative risk assessments lend themselves to numerical characterizations of the uncertainty attending risks. Deterministic risk characterizations can be supplemented by offering high/low, optimistic/pessimistic, or more formal statistical confidence interval estimates of decision criteria and risks estimated in the assessment. Using interval estimates for uncertain inputs and tracking their impact on critical outputs is a feasible way to identify and communicate what is most important. In probabilistic risk assessment, the challenges of communication are greater, because although there is usually more useful information, it is quantitatively complex and problematic for many risk managers and stakeholders who lack training in interpreting and understanding probabilistic data. The basic problem in risk assessment is that our data are incomplete and we are uncertain about many things. None of this absolves us of the need to make decisions, however. Risk assessment is a process through which complex, incomplete, uncertain, and often contradictory evidence and scientific information are made useful for decision making (NRC, 1983). As a decision-support framework, risk assessment fills the gap between the available evidence and the RMOs being considered to respond to the risks identified. Risk managers must understand those gaps, how they were bridged, and their significance for decision making. It is the assessor's job to explain all of this to them.

## 4.4.8   Document the process

Risk assessment is initiated to support decision making that solves problems and realizes opportunities. Substantial resources are dedicated to risk assessment, and it is essential that we carefully and effectively document its findings. It is equally important to document the basis for the risk management actions taken or not taken. Think of documentation as a set of different communications that authenticate and support the results of the risk management activity. The hope is that risk management decisions will be directly linked to the evidence found in the risk assessment documentation.

Assessors are well advised to document the assessment process as it progresses rather than to wait until it has been finished to write up a report. Risk assessment generally progresses in an iterative fashion. Our understanding of problems evolves as the assessment progresses. Analysis is refined as data gaps are filled and models are built. Numerous people will be involved at many points along the way. It is often easier to have assessors document their findings as they go, revising them as new data and analysis warrant.

---

**TELLING YOUR STORY**

Storytelling is underestimated as an effective communication skill. Stop listing facts and dumping data into reports and tell a simple story well. We all remember engaging stories from our childhood and they had three key elements in common:

An engaging beginning...once upon a time;
An interesting middle...consider a talking mirror;
A satisfying ending...they all lived happily ever after.

Tell the story by structuring the facts so they have a narrative quality. Let your documentation be a journey with a narrative theme. Good stories are simple, let the facts speak for themselves.

---

Documentation need not be restricted to a written report. Nontraditional risk assessment documentation methods might include:

- Interactive websites
- Interactive digital media
- Video reports
- Workshops
- Chat rooms

- Wikis
- Discussion groups
- Electronic files
- Training in the use of the risk assessment model
- Live online briefings
- Page limits on written documents

Identify your audience and choose a suitable documentation format.

## 4.5    Risk assessment models

The generic risk assessment tasks you've been reading about have been standardized for a variety of applications and communities of practice (CoP). The food-safety community, for example, has been aggressive in trying to harmonize risk assessment methods in part to facilitate international trade. They, like other CoPs, have promulgated models for use by their constituents. A few of these models are presented in this section to illustrate the diverse range of ways in which these rather generic risk assessment activities are being formalized for specific applications. The details of the model are less important than the overarching point that risk assessors exercise a great deal of latitude in the specific ways they do risk assessments.

The *Codex Alimentarius* represents the international food-safety community. They employ a familiar risk assessment model, shown in Figure 4.7. Within or alongside of this framework, CoPs have developed distinctive models and methodologies for different hazards like food-additive chemicals, pesticides, microbiological hazards, food nutrients, antimicrobial resistance, and genetically modified organisms.

Chemical food additives are evaluated using a safety assessment, which on the surface looks quite different from the generic model of this chapter. Its six steps comprise the following: test toxicity, identify NOAEL, choose a safety factor, calculate the ADI, calculate the EDI, and characterize the risk with the ratio EDI/ADI.

A conceptual application of the model is presented in Figure 4.8. Toxicity studies, most often based on animal data, are used to identify a level of exposure to a chemical, usually measured in a lifetime dose that causes no adverse effects. This is equivalent to a hazard characterization. In the example in Figure 4.8, this level is 5 mg per kg of body weight daily for a lifetime.

To extrapolate from animal studies and their typically high doses to humans and their typically low doses, an uncertainty factor (in the example, 100) is used to identify an ADI. Thus, a NOAEL of 5 mg/kg/day/lifetime divided by 100 yields an ADI of 0.05 mg/kg/day/lifetime.

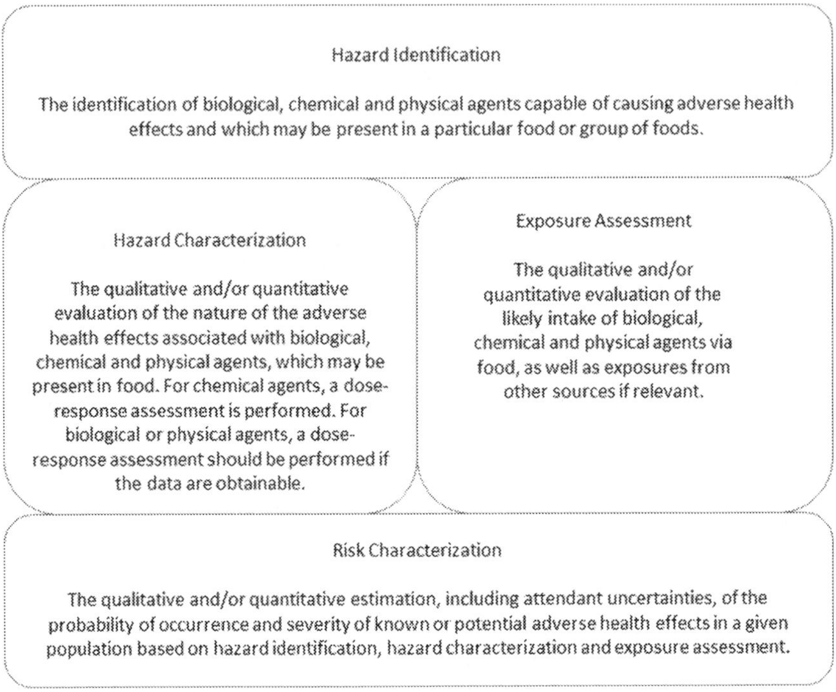

Hazard Identification

The identification of biological, chemical and physical agents capable of causing adverse health effects and which may be present in a particular food or group of foods.

Hazard Characterization

The qualitative and/or quantitative evaluation of the nature of the adverse health effects associated with biological, chemical and physical agents, which may be present in food. For chemical agents, a dose-response assessment is performed. For biological or physical agents, a dose-response assessment should be performed if the data are obtainable.

Exposure Assessment

The qualitative and/or quantitative evaluation of the likely intake of biological, chemical and physical agents via food, as well as exposures from other sources if relevant.

Risk Characterization

The qualitative and/or quantitative estimation, including attendant uncertainties, of the probability of occurrence and severity of known or potential adverse health effects in a given population based on hazard identification, hazard characterization and exposure assessment.

*Figure 4.7* Generic *Codex* description of the risk assessment components. (From Food and Agricultural Organization. 2006. United Nations. FAO Food and Nutrition Paper 87. *Food safety risk analysis: A guide for national food safety authorities.* Rome, Italy: FAO.)

A survey of consumption behavior yields the daily consumption of the additive for a high-end consumer, say the 90th percentile consumer of this additive, and this is used as the EDI. This constitutes the exposure assessment. The risk characterization is completed by simply comparing the EDI to the ADI. There is no effort to explicitly identify the likelihood of an adverse outcome in this assessment model.

Pesticide chemical risks are somewhat similar, although the language changes a little:

- Identify pesticide residue of interest
- Undertake toxicity studies of substance if needed
- Determine the NOAEL
- Select a safety factor or uncertainty factor to extrapolate results from animals to humans

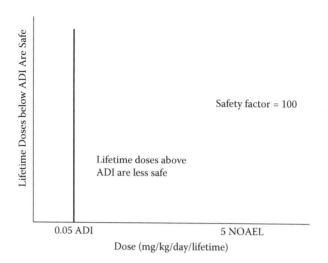

*Figure 4.8* Representation of the food-additive safety assessment model.

- Calculate the ADI
- Identify a suitable index of residue levels to predict residue intake—usually the maximum residue limit (MRL)
- Estimate the dietary intake of the residue (exposure assessment)
- Compare exposure to ADI (when exposure exceeds ADI, some sort of risk mitigation is required)

Note that although the language differs in each, they all exhibit elements of the previously described generic process. The hazard is identified; the consequences and likelihoods (or exposures) are assessed; and it is all pulled together in some sort of characterization of the risk.

Antimicrobial-resistant risk assessment is used to evaluate the safety of new animal drugs with respect to concerns for human health. Exposing bacteria in animals to antimicrobial drugs could increase the number of resistant bacteria to the point where it reduces the efficacy of antimicrobial drugs prescribed for human health. This model, shown in Figure 4.9 and taken from FDA Guidance Document 152 (FDA, 2003), suggests a qualitative approach for identifying new drugs as potentially high, medium, or low risks for human health.

Food safety is not the only CoP to have developed standardized mental models to guide thinking about risk assessment. The EPA (1998) developed the model shown in Figure 4.10 for ecological risk assessment. Note that it differs from the four-step definition of the "Red Book" but has clear roots in that model as well. The "Red Book" model was developed principally

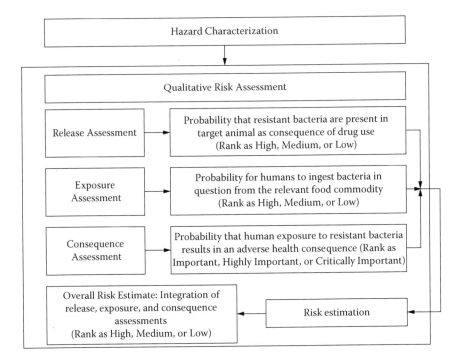

***Figure 4.9*** Components of a qualitative antimicrobial-resistance risk assessment. (From Food and Drug Administration. 2003. *Guidance for industry evaluating the safety of antimicrobial new animal drugs with regard to their microbiological effects on bacteria of human health concern.* No. 152. Rockville, MD: Center for Veterinary Medicine. http:// www.fda.gov/downloads/AnimalVeterinary/GuidanceComplianceEnforcement/ GuidanceforIndustry/UCM052519.pdf.)

for assessing human health risks due to chemicals in the environment. The ecological model expands the notion of hazards to include a broad class of stressors and it includes adverse effects on ecosystems. It has three main steps: problem formulation, analysis, and risk characterization.

Hazards are identified as stressors in problem formulation. The analysis step is divided into characterizations of exposure and ecological effects, the latter of which is evocative of the hazard characterization step. The risk characterization step serves the familiar purpose. The point here is that although the models vary in their language and details, they remain firmly committed to the principles articulated in the tasks identified earlier in this chapter.

If you search Internet images using the phrase "risk assessment model," you'll see thousands of different models in millions of hits. Many risk assessment problems are so unique that they cannot be usefully fit to any of the existing mental models for risk assessment. It is always wise to

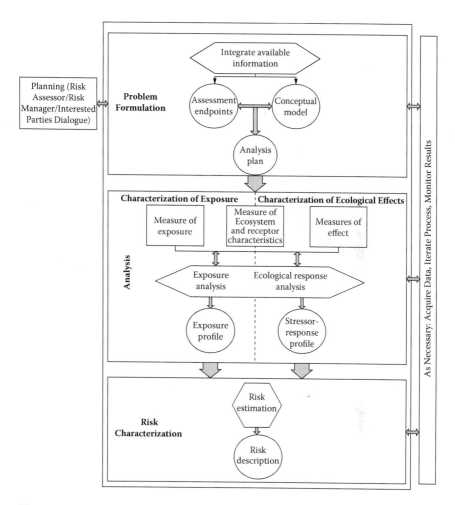

*Figure 4.10* Ecological risk assessment framework, with an expanded view of each phase. (From Environmental Protection Agency. 1998. *Federal Register* 63 (93): 26846–26924.)

familiarize yourself with any standardized assessment models used by your CoP. More importantly, you should always feel free to adapt these models or to develop your own mental model when it suits your decision-making needs to do so. If you flounder at times, keep coming back to the four informal questions: What can go wrong? What are the consequences? How can it happen? How likely is it? Find a way to ask and answer these questions and you will be doing risk assessment, formal model or not.

Very often, an organization has a model with a well-established structure. Consider the model in Table 4.1, which is used to estimate the

*Table 4.1* Channel modification dredging cost estimate

| Account code | Description | Quantity | Unit[a] | Unit price | Amount |
|---|---|---|---|---|---|
| 01 | Lands and damages | 0 | LS | — | — |
| 02 | Relocations | | | | |
| | Lower 20 pipeline, 653 + 00 | 427 | LF | $843.66 | $359,979 |
| | Remove 8″ pipeline, 678 + 00 | 986 | LF | $47.85 | $47,197 |
| 02 | *Total—relocations* | | | | *$407,176* |
| 06 | Fish and wildlife facilities (mitigation) | | | | |
| | Oyster reef creation | 0 | ACR | — | — |
| 06 | *Total—fish and wildlife facilities (mitigation)* | | | | — |
| 12 | Navigation, ports, and harbors | | | | |
| | Mobe and demobe | 1 | LS | $500,000 | $500,000 |
| | Pipeline dredging, Reach 1 | 576,107.00 | CY | $2.43 | $1,398,788 |
| | Pipeline dredging, Reach 2 | 1,161,626.68 | CY | $2.76 | $3,209,691 |
| | Pipeline dredging, Reach 3A | 1,532,227.12 | CY | $3.72 | $5,693,450 |
| | Pipeline dredging, Reach 3B | 708,252.02 | CY | $2.89 | $2,049,398 |
| | Scour pad, Reach 1 | 16,484 | SY | $16.62 | $273,906 |
| | Geotubes, 30′, Reach 1 | 1,345 | LF | $221.03 | $297,192 |
| | Geotubes, 45′, Reach 1 | 4,601 | LF | $291.00 | $1,338,995 |
| | Scour pad, Reach 3 | 39,059 | SY | $16.62 | $649,029 |
| | Geotubes, 45′, Reach 3 | 13,848 | LF | $291.00 | $4,029,879 |
| 12 | *Total—navigation, ports, and harbors Subtotal* | | | | *$19,440,328* |
| 30 | Engineering and design | 8% | | | $1,587,800 |
| 31 | Construction management | 6% | | | $1,190,850 |
| | *Total project cost* | | | | *$22,626,154* |

[a] LF = linear feet; LS = lump sum; CY = cubic yards; SY = square yards, ACR = acres.

costs of a dredging project that includes marsh creation for disposal of the dredged material. It is not difficult to imagine that risk managers may be concerned with the risk of a cost overrun. There is no need here to develop a conceptual model. In this instance, the structure of the model is well established and we need only reach into the risk assessors' toolbox for the appropriate techniques for assessing this risk using our four informal questions. For now, it is sufficient to understand that there is a large class of problems that require no specific risk assessment model. Often it is sufficient to pay appropriate attention to the uncertainty that has always been present in our work. In many instances, risk assessment can mean doing what you have always done, with the exception of paying close attention to the things you do not know. Using the generic risk assessment activities described here should provide you with a serviceable model when a formal one is not available.

## 4.6   Risk assessment methods

Any self-contained systematic procedure conducted as part of a risk assessment is a risk assessment method (Covello and Merkhofer, 1993). These methods are conveniently divided into qualitative and quantitative methods. There has been a misperception on the parts of some and a bias on the parts of others who have suggested that qualitative risk assessment is not a valid form of risk assessment. I think it fair to say that quantitative risk assessment is preferred whenever there are data adequate to support it. It is equally fair to say that qualitative risk assessment is a valid and valuable form of risk assessment. Quantitative assessments use numerical expressions to characterize the risks; qualitative assessments do not.

### 4.6.1   Qualitative risk assessment

The fundamental need is to manage risk intentionally and to do that better than has been done in the past. Quantitative risk assessment is not always possible or necessary, so qualitative risk assessment is often a viable and valuable option. It is especially useful:

- For routine noncontroversial tasks
- When consistency and transparency in handling risk are desired
- When theory, data, time, or expertise are limited
- When dealing with broadly defined problems where quantitative risk assessment is impractical

A qualitative risk assessment process compiles, combines, and presents evidence to support a nonnumerical estimate and description of a risk. Numerical data and analysis may be part of the input to a qualitative risk assessment, but they are not part of the risk characterization output. Qualitative assessment produces a descriptive or categorical treatment of risk information. It is a formal, organized, reproducible, and flexible method based on science and sound evidence that produces consistent descriptions of risk that are easy to explain to others. Its value stems from its ability to support risk management decision making. If you can answer the risk manager's questions adequately and describe the risk in a narrative or categorically, then a qualitative assessment is sufficient. Uncertainty in qualitative assessments is generally addressed through descriptive narratives.

### 4.6.2   Quantitative risk assessment

Quantitative risk assessment relies on numerical expressions of risk in the risk characterization. Numerical measures of risk are generally more informative than qualitative estimates. When the data and resources are sufficient, a quantitative assessment is preferred, except where the risk manager's questions can be adequately answered in a narrative or categorical fashion.

Quantitative assessments can be deterministic or probabilistic. Deterministic assessments produce point estimates of risks. Probabilistic assessments rely on probability distributions and probability statements to estimate risks. The choice depends on the risk manager's questions, available data, the nature of the uncertainties, the skills of the assessors, the effectiveness of outputs in informing and supporting decision makers, and the number and robustness of the assumptions made in the assessment.

Generally, quantitative risk characterizations address risk management questions at a finer level of detail and resolution than a qualitative risk assessment. This greater detail usually introduces a more sophisticated treatment of the uncertainty in the risk characterization than is found with qualitative assessment.

## 4.7   Summary and look forward

Risk assessment is where the evidence is gathered. It is the primary place where we separate what we know from what we do not know and then deal intentionally with those things we do not know. It is where we get the right science focused into the analysis and take pains to get that science right.

In general terms, risk assessment is the work you must do to answer four informal questions. What can go wrong? What are the consequences? How can it happen? How likely is it? The four primary steps that comprise a risk assessment and answer these questions are: identify the hazards and opportunities, assess the consequences, assess the likelihood, and characterize the risk. There are any number of application-specific refinements of these notions in widespread use. Recurring kinds of problems lend themselves well to the development of standardized approaches to assessing these risks.

In the best practice of risk assessment, risk managers will identify specific questions they want the risk assessment to answer. Risk assessors answer these questions and characterize the uncertainty in their assessment in ways that support risk-informed decision making. The answers to these questions can be provided in a qualitative or a quantitative manner, depending on the needs of the risk management activity.

Estimating and describing risks in the risk assessment is the critical analytical step in risk analysis. But if we are not able to communicate this often-complex information to risk managers, stakeholders, and the public, all will have been for naught. The next chapter addresses the risk communication component of risk analysis. Until relatively recently, risk communication has been treated like the stepchild of risk analysis, too often an afterthought or an add-on. More recently, it has begun to receive more of the attention it rightfully deserves.

## References

Covello, V.T., and M.W. Merkhofer. 1993. *Risk assessment methods: Approaches for assessing health and environmental risks.* New York: Plenum Press.

Covello, V.T., and J. Mumpower. 1985. Risk analysis and risk management: An historical perspective. *Risk Analysis* 5 (2): 103–119.

Cox, L.A., Jr. 2002. *Risk analysis foundations, models, and methods.* Boston: Kluwer Academic.

Environmental Protection Agency (EPA). 1998. *Guidelines for ecological risk assessment.* EPA/630/R-95/002F. *Federal Register* 63 (93): 26846–26924.

Food and Agricultural Organization (FAO). 2006. United Nations. FAO Food and Nutrition Paper 87. *Food safety risk analysis: A guide for national food safety authorities.* Rome, Italy: FAO.

Food and Agricultural Organization and World Health Organization (FAO/WHO). 2004. United Nations. *Codex Alimentarius Commission, procedural manual.* 14th ed. Rome, Italy: FAO.

Food and Drug Administration (FDA). 2003. *Guidance for industry evaluating the safety of antimicrobial new animal drugs with regard to their microbiological effects on bacteria of human health concern.* No. 152. Rockville, MD: Center for Veterinary Medicine. http://www.fda.gov/downloads/AnimalVeterinary/GuidanceComplianceEnforcement/GuidanceforIndustry/UCM052519.pdf.

Food and Drug Administration (FDA). 2005. *Quantitative risk assessment on the public health impact of pathogenic Vibrio parahaemolyticus in raw oysters.* College Park, MD: Center for Food Safety and Applied Nutrition. http://www.fda.gov/Food/ScienceResearch/ResearchAreas/RiskAssessmentSafetyAssessment/ucm050421.htm.

International Programme on Chemical Safety (IPCS). 2008. *Uncertainty and data quality in exposure assessment, part 1 and part 2.* Geneva, Switzerland: World Health Organization.

International Organization of Standardization (ISO). 2009. *Risk management— principles and guidelines.* Geneva, Switzerland: International Organization of Standardization.

National Research Council (NRC). 1983. Committee on the Institutional Means for Assessment of Risks to Public Health. *Risk assessment in the federal government: Managing the process.* Washington, DC: National Academies Press.

National Research Council (NRC). 1994. Committee on Risk Assessment of Hazardous Air Pollutants. *Science and judgment in risk assessment.* Washington DC: National Academies Press.

National Research Council (NRC). 1996. Committee on Risk Characterization. *Understanding risk: Informing decisions in a democratic society.* Washington, DC: National Academies Press.

Presidential/Congressional Commission on Risk Assessment and Risk Management. 1997a. "Framework for environmental health risk management." Final report, vol. 1. Washington, DC: www.riskworld.com. http://riskworld.com/nreports/1997/risk-rpt/pdf/EPAJAN.PDF.

Presidential/Congressional Commission on Risk Assessment and Risk Management. 1997b. "Framework for environmental health risk management." Final report, vol. 2. Washington, DC: www.riskworld.com. http://riskworld.com/nreports/1997/risk-rpt/volume2/pdf/v2epa.pdf.

Toffler, A. 1990. *Powershift: Knowledge, Wealth and Violence at the Edge of the 21st Century.* New York: Bantam Books.

# chapter five

---

# Risk communication

## 5.1 Introduction

Risk communication is one of the three components of risk analysis. It is now prominently featured in most risk analysis models. Let me summarize the history of risk analysis in three nonscientific figures, seen in Figure 5.1.

An ideal balance of the three risk analysis tasks is shown in the figure on the bottom left. Here, the three tasks are coequal, with modest overlap but functional integrity. Not so long ago, risk analysis might have been described by the figure on the top left. Risk assessment was the tail wagging the dog. Risk management was an afterthought, and risk communication was scarcely on the horizon. In fact, there were many models of risk analysis that did not even mention it! Risk communication was for years the bastard child of risk analysis, seldom talked about and often ignored or treated poorly. Other than a few devoted adherents, it struggled for any recognition at all.

In the recent past, risk management has grown in importance and stature, and the descriptive model might be that shown on the top right of Figure 5.1. While risk management came of age and now guides risk assessment, risk communication too often remained the weak link in actual practice. That always comes at a cost. Because of those costs, risk communication is finally coming into its own, and it is now increasingly recognized in models and, more importantly, by organizations as being at least as important as the assessment and management tasks. Like the other components, its definition is difficult to pin down in words that will satisfy everyone. The term means different things to different people, and a wide variety of definitions can be found in the literature and organizational guidance of different institutions.

Despite the variations in definitions, there is a growing consensus on a set of core principles for risk communication that include the following:

- It is an interactive exchange of information and opinion
- It takes place throughout the risk analysis process
- It concerns risk, risk-related factors, and risk perceptions
- It involves risk assessors and risk managers as well as affected groups and individuals and interested parties
- It includes an explanation of the risk, an explanation of the risk assessment, and the basis for the risk management decision

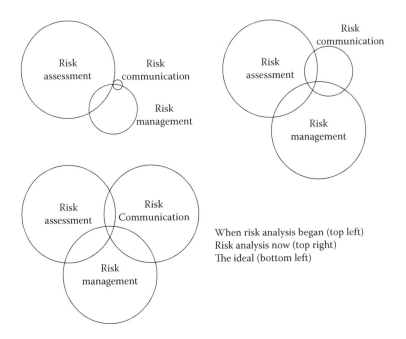

*Figure 5.1* The role of risk communication in risk analysis.

There are many reasons to communicate about risks, including the goals of achieving a consensus understanding of the magnitude of the risk and developing credible and acceptable risk management responses. Risk communication improves understanding of the risk and risk management options (RMOs). It enhances trust and confidence in the decision-making process and promotes the participation and involvement of interested parties. Done well, it can strengthen working relationships among stakeholders.

Risk communication is needed to explain actions to avoid or take risks, and it is needed to explain the rationale for the chosen RMO. The effectiveness and workings of a specific option need to be communicated to people so they understand their own risk management responsibilities and know what actions they must take to reduce the risk. The benefits of an RMO as well as the costs of managing the risk and who will bear them, are additional information to be conveyed to interested parties. Risk communication needs to pay special attention to describing the risks that remain after the RMO is implemented. The uncertainty that could affect the magnitude of the risk or the efficacy of the RMO must be carefully communicated to stakeholders and the public. This should include the weaknesses, limitations of, or inaccuracies in the available evidence. It should also include the important assumptions on which risk estimates are based so that stakeholders can understand the sensitivity of both risk estimates and the efficacy of an

RMO to changes in those assumptions and how those changes can affect risk management decisions. It should include a description of the range of outcomes that can result from a risk management decision.

Risk communication does not require everyone to reach a consensus or an agreement. Neither is it intended to get everybody on the "same page." It is, however, about providing people with meaningful opportunities for input before decisions are made and for feedback as evidence is accumulated. It is about listening to and understanding people's concerns so they can be considered in decision making and so the public will respect the process even if they disagree with some of its decisions and outcomes.

Risk communication theory and practice are well documented in a very rich risk communications literature. For example, see the works by Chess and Hance (1994), Chess et al. (1989), Covello (2002), Covello and Allen (1988), Covello and Cohrssen (1989), Covello and Merkhofer (1993), Covello and Mumpower (1985), Covello and Sandman (2001), Covello et al. (1988, 1989, 2001), Fischhoff (1986, 1995), Fischoff et al. (1978), Hance et al. (1990), Johnson and Covello (1987), Krimsky and Plough (1988), Sandman (1987, 1989, 1999, 2004, 2010a, 2010b, 2010c), Sandman and Lanard (2003, 2005), Slovic (1987), Slovic et al. (1980, 1990), and others presented in the references at the end of this chapter. How one frames the risk communication component for the purposes of risk analysis is of some importance because the scope and role of risk communication is rapidly advancing. To some, the risk communication component is relatively narrow and focuses on risk and crisis communication. I think this is far too narrow a definition, even while recognizing its adequacy for many situations. A more proactive expanded view of risk communication is provided in Figure 5.2.

Risk communication can first be split into internal and external tasks. Internal risk communication takes place within the risk analysis team. It begins with the coordination between the assessors and managers that has been described in the previous two chapters. This aspect of risk communication is arguably little different from the kind of good organizational communication that is part of any effective organization's management philosophy. I make a distinction because it involves communicating about uncertainty and talking about what we do not know is not something many organizations do well. The coordination is ongoing throughout a risk management activity.

Developing and conducting an effective risk communication process is not something that happens by accident. Good risk communication cannot be an afterthought or an add-on. Neither is it a hypodermic needle injection into the activity at prescribed or periodic points in time. It needs to be a dynamic ongoing process. To be so, it must be designed.

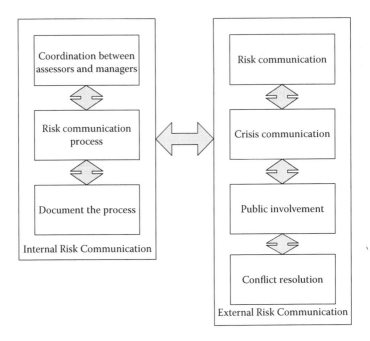

*Figure 5.2* Components of the internal and external risk communication tasks.

**BEST PRACTICES FOR RISK COMMUNICATION**

1. Infuse risk communication into policy decisions.
2. Treat risk communication as a process.
3. Account for the uncertainty inherent in risk.
4. Design risk messages to be culturally sensitive.
5. Acknowledge diverse levels of risk tolerance.
6. Involve the public in dialogue about risk.
7. Present risk messages with honesty.
8. Meet risk perception needs by remaining open and accessible to the public.
9. Collaborate and coordinate about risk with credible information sources.

**Source: Effective Risk Communication:
A Message-Centered Approach
(Sellnow et al., 2009)**

Documenting the process is usually described (including in this book) as a management or assessment process, and it is. There is little that is more fundamental to the internal risk communication process, however, than documenting the results of the activity and the decisions made from them. These internal risk communication tasks are often given little attention in the literature, which tends to favor the external risk communication processes shown on the right side of Figure 5.2.

Most texts on risk communication focus on risk and crisis communication, as will this chapter. Nonetheless, my work with risk analysis organizations around the world suggests that there is a growing recognition of the need to expand the public's role in the risk analysis process. It makes sense to me to expand the definition of risk communication activities to include public-involvement and, in some cases, conflict-resolution activities; however, I am not sure there is anything close to a consensus on that idea just yet.

The chapter begins with definitions. It then briefly considers the three internal risk communication tasks of Figure 5.2. It moves into the area of external risk communications and begins a discussion of risk and crisis communications by considering the important distinction between the hazard and outrage dimensions of risk, which interact to define very distinct risk communication strategies. Risk perceptions, the next topic, are important for understanding the disconnect between producers and consumers of risk information.

Just as strategies for risk communication vary, so do the audiences for these strategies. The next discussion covers the importance of knowing the psychographic characteristics of the audiences for your communications. A basic communication model is presented to lay the framework for emphasizing the role of stress in risk communication, followed by an introduction to the three M's of risk communication. Some of the critical differences between crisis and risk communication are considered before the chapter turns to the challenge of explaining risk to nonexperts. This leads into a discussion about explaining uncertainty, a task as critical to risk assessors and risk managers as it is to risk communicators. The chapter ends with a short consideration of public involvement and conflict resolution.

To prepare you for what follows, I offer two keywords. The keyword for the internal risk communication task is uncertainty. The keyword for the external risk communication task is emotion. Get a handle on how to communicate uncertainty to people who are feeling strong emotions and the efficacy of your risk communication efforts will improve dramatically.

## 5.2   Definitions

No one formal definition of risk communication will meet the needs of all practitioners of risk communication. The *Codex Alimentarius* offers a definition that is quite expansive. It says risk communication is: "The interactive exchange of information and opinions throughout the risk analysis process concerning risk, risk-related factors and risk perceptions, among risk assessors, risk managers, consumers, industry, the academic community and other interested parties, including the explanation of risk assessment findings and the basis of risk management decisions" (FAO, 2004).

---

### COMMUNICATING WITH THE PUBLIC:
### 10 QUESTIONS TO ASK

1. Why are we communicating?
2. Who is our audience?
3. What do our audiences want to know?
4. What do we want to get across?
5. How will we communicate?
6. How will we listen?
7. How will we respond?
8. Who will carry out the plans? When?
9. What problems or barriers have we planned for?
10. Have we succeeded?

**Source: Chess and Hance (1994)**

---

A shorter and simpler definition from the U.S. Department of Agriculture is also useful. Risk communication is "an open, two-way exchange of information and opinion about risk leading to better understanding and better risk management decisions" (University of Minnesota, 2006). An informal definition is implicitly offered by the 10 questions shown in the text box. Risk communication is the work you have to do to answer those 10 questions.

## 5.3    Internal risk communication

### 5.3.1    Coordination between assessors and managers

The internal risk communication task is essential to ensure effective interaction between managers and assessors. Three rules of thumb are suggested for this task for the managers and assessors:

- Collaborate early
- Coordinate often
- Cooperate always

Early risk analysis experience and, subsequently, models showed the need to separate the roles of managers and assessors. In their zeal to ensure the integrity of the science-based foundation of risk analysis, some early practitioners were somewhat manic about this separation and stretched it almost to the point of no contact. That is most emphatically not best practice. Although the integrity of the science needs to be relentlessly protected, managers and assessors need to interact constantly throughout the risk analysis process despite the fact that they have very clear and different individual responsibilities.

Referring to the risk management activities described in Chapter 3, the extent of the interaction between risk assessors and risk managers is suggested below using a scale of no, minimal, moderate, and maximum interaction based on the author's experience.

1. Problem identification
   a.  Problem recognition: *moderate interaction*
   b.  Problem acceptance: *no interaction*
   c.  Problem definition: *maximum interaction*
2. Risk estimation
   a.  Establish risk analysis process: *minimal interaction*
   b.  Develop a risk profile: *maximum interaction*
   c.  Establish risk management objectives: *moderate interaction*
   d.  Decide on the need for risk assessment: *no interaction*
   e.  Request information: *moderate interaction*
   f.  Initiate risk assessment: *moderate interaction*
   g.  Coordinate the conduct of the assessment: *moderate interaction*
   h.  Consider the results of the assessment: *maximum interaction*
3. Risk evaluation
   a.  Is the risk acceptable: *no interaction*
   b.  Establish tolerable level of risk: *moderate interaction*
   c.  Risk management strategies: *maximum interaction*
4. Risk control
   a.  Formulating risk management options (RMOs): *maximum interaction*
   b.  Evaluating RMOs: *moderate interaction*
   c.  Comparing RMOs: *moderate interaction*
   d.  Making a decision: *no interaction*
   e.  Identifying decision outcomes: *moderate interaction*
   f.  Implementing the decision: *no interaction*
5. Monitoring
   a.  Monitor: *moderate interaction*
   b.  Evaluate: *moderate interaction*
   c.  Modify: *moderate interaction*

Turning to the risk assessment activities of Chapter 4 and using the same subjective scale, the author's judgments are:

1. Understand the question(s): *maximum interaction*
2. Identify the source of the risk: *moderate interaction*
3. Consequence assessment: *no interaction*
4. Likelihood assessment: *no interaction*
5. Risk characterization: *no interaction*
6. Assess effectiveness of RMOs: *moderate interaction*
7. Communicate uncertainty: *maximum interaction*
8. Document the process: *moderate interaction*

Some of the most critical points of interaction occur at the beginning and end of the risk management activity. Identifying problems, objectives, and the initial list of questions together are essential early interactions, as is preparing a risk profile. These tasks will also provide stakeholders with opportunities for input and feedback in best-practice risk communication.

Revising the risk assessment questions together, when necessary, is an especially important interaction. This clarifies the information needs of the risk managers and is an essential step in managing the expectations of both managers and assessors. Interaction is clearly needed to set reasonable assessment schedules, budgets, and milestones together. The two parties are to do their own jobs, but they should brief each other often. After the risk assessment is completed, understanding the results of the assessment and significant uncertainties together are critical interactions. Interaction continues, but the manager's role increases relative to the assessor's after the assessment is completed. The risk manager's role is preeminent when asking, "Is the current level of risk acceptable" or "What level of risk is tolerable?"

Managers and assessors should formulate risk management options together. They also need to coordinate the evaluation of options together to ensure that managers have the information they need to decide which measures are best. This may happen before, during, or after the risk assessment. Assessors are responsible for the analytical work in the evaluation of RMOs, while risk managers do the deliberating in these tasks.

To a great extent, this internal communication task is just good organizational management. It is not unique to risk analysis. What is somewhat unique in risk analysis is the role of communicating effectively about those things that are uncertain and potentially important for decision making.

## 5.3.2 Risk communication process

Designing the external risk communication process, outlined in the remainder of this chapter, is a critical part of the risk analysis team's internal communications task. Creighton's (2005) book on public participation provides an excellent blueprint for those looking to provide a larger and more active role for the public. A narrower and more traditional risk communication program can be designed following the templates in risk communication handbooks like those of Lundgren and McMakin (2009) and Heath and O'Hair (2009).

## 5.3.3 Documenting the process

Telling the story of the risk management process and the risk assessment is also an important part of the internal risk communication task. The decision process must be carefully documented to provide a defensible rationale for actions taken or not taken as a result of the risk analysis process. Risk managers, ideally with the assistance of risk communication experts, should carefully plan the documentation of the process.

# 5.4 External risk communication

The external communication tasks generally describe how the risk analysis team (managers, assessors, and communicators) interacts with their various publics and external stakeholders. These interactions can overlap with the internal tasks, as may be the case for identifying problems and objectives as well as preparing the risk profile and the initial list of questions, when external input is likely to be important. The extent to which this may happen will depend on how involved the public is in the risk management activity. Four broad tasks have been identified as part of the external risk communication process. These are:

- Risk communication
- Crisis communication
- Public involvement
- Conflict resolution

An external communication program will not always require all four elements. For the purposes of the current discussion, we will focus narrowly on a more traditional risk communication process and will return to considerations of public involvement and conflict resolution at the end of the chapter.

## GOALS OF RISK COMMUNICATION

1. Promote awareness and understanding of the specific issues under consideration during the risk analysis process, by all participants.
2. Promote consistency and transparency in arriving at and implementing risk management decisions.
3. Provide a sound basis for understanding the risk management decisions proposed or implemented.
4. Improve the overall effectiveness and efficiency of the risk analysis process.
5. Contribute to the development and delivery of effective information and education programs, when they are selected as risk management options.
6. Foster public trust and confidence in the safety of the food supply.
7. Strengthen the working relationships and mutual respect among all participants.
8. Promote the appropriate involvement of all interested parties in the risk communication process.
9. Exchange information on the knowledge, attitudes, values, practices, and perceptions of interested parties concerning risks associated with food and related topics.

**Source: The Application of Risk Communication to Food Standards and Safety Matters, a Joint FAO/WHO Expert Consultation (UN, 1998)**

The external risk communication process can have many different goals. Three reasonably common, if not universal, generic goals (Food Insight, 2010)[*] are:

1. Tailor communication so it takes into account the emotional response to an event.
2. Empower the audience to make informed decisions.
3. Prevent negative behavior and encourage constructive responses to crisis or danger.

[*] I would like to acknowledge the Food Insight materials, sponsored by the International Food Information Council Foundation, as a major source of information for much of the discussion in Section 5.4 of this chapter.

Unlike the basic unidirectional, "We tell them what we did," communication model, risk communication is two-way (listening and speaking) and multidirectional. It uses multiple sources of communication, and it actively involves the audience as an information source. Risk analysts can learn from individuals, communities, and organizations.

The desired outcomes of effective risk communication will vary from problem to problem, but there are some generic outcomes that recur with regularity. First, it can decrease deaths, illness, injury, and other adverse consequences of risks by informing people and changing behaviors. Alternatively, it can increase the positive outcomes of opportunities. It fosters informed decision making concerning risk and empowers people through useful and timely information to make their own informed decisions. It prevents the misallocation and wasting of resources and keeps decision makers well informed. Good risk communication builds support for risk management options and can aid the successful implementation of an RMO. It also can counter or correct rumors.

Risk communication is not spinning a situation to control the public's reaction, nor is it public relations or damage control. It is more than how to write a press release or how to give a media interview. It is not always intended to make people "feel better" or to reduce their fear. It is multidirectional communication among communicators, publics, and stakeholders that considers human perceptions of risk as well as the science-based assessment of risk. It includes activities before, during, and after an event. It is during these activities that risk communication can broaden to include public involvement. Risk communication is an integral part of an emergency response plan. Aware of the many dimensions of risk communication, let us drill down a little deeper to understand it better.

## 5.4.1    Risk and crisis communication

This section covers the first two elements of the external risk communication task. The discussion begins with some important background information that addresses the dimensions and perceptions of risk before it turns to the importance of knowing and engaging one's audiences. The value of psychographic information is considered as a lead-in to the consideration of risk, stress, and the communication model. The three M's of risk communication are then discussed. Risk and crisis communication are juxtaposed for distinction, and then the discussion turns to the challenges of explaining risk and uncertainty to nonexperts.

### 5.4.1.1   Risk dimensions

Virtually everything we do involves risk, and zero risk is unachievable in both our personal and professional lives. Risk communication is complicated by the fact that people interpret risk in very different ways, especially experts and the public. Risk involves both facts and feelings, and these competing dimensions of risk—the objective vs. the subjective—give rise to some unique communication challenges.

---

### HAZARD AND OUTRAGE

Let's divide the "risk" that people are worried about into two components. The technical side of the risk focuses on the magnitude and probability of undesirable outcomes: an increase in the cancer rate, a catastrophic accident, dead fish in the river, or a decline in property values. Call all this "hazard."

The nontechnical side of the risk focuses on everything negative about the situation itself, as opposed to those outcomes. Is it voluntary or coerced, familiar or exotic, dreaded or not dreaded? Are you trustworthy or untrustworthy, responsive or unresponsive? Call all this "outrage."

**Source: Sandman (1999)**

---

Peter Sandman (1999) describes these two elements of risk as hazard and outrage (see text box). These two elements shape the perceptions of risk. In general, hazard (the something that can go wrong, its factual consequences, and the likelihood of it happening) is what the assessors and scientists are primarily concerned with. Experts think about these hazards, and they know things that others do not. Predictive microbiologists know the conditions under which a pathogen may grow or die off. Engineers understand the hydrographs of rivers. Financial advisers understand the subtle details of their derivatives. Toxicologists know how much of a chemical is toxic. Most of the rest of us do not know these things.

The public is concerned less with the science, numbers, and facts of the risk and more with the personal and social context of the risk. The public feels things about the risks, and they believe things to be true or not, often without respect to the facts of a situation. The public is less concerned with the details of the probabilities than they are with a subjective evaluation of the relative importance of what might be lost. They do not care about pathogen growth; they care that their daughter got sick. They could care less about the hydrograph; they do care that their first floor was damaged by the flood. The details of the derivatives are of less interest than the college fund that was lost.

These two distinct dimensions of a risk can lead to a disconnect between the scientist/risk professional and the public. Scientists tend to focus on what they know and think, while the public focuses on what they feel and believe. Both dimensions of a risk are important, but for different reasons. They are very different aspects of a risk. Sometimes, the public worries when perhaps the scientists would say they shouldn't, for example, about irradiated foods. Other times they may not worry about things scientists think they should be worried about, for example, the oncoming hurricane.

Risk communication that is based wholly on explaining the facts of the risk may well miss the greater concerns of the public, which tend to be the social context and personal meaning of the risk. There is a whole lot more to risk communication than explaining the results of your risk assessment. This disconnect between producers (scientists) and consumers (the public) of risk information gives rise to four kinds of risk communication strategies (adapted from Sandman and Lanard, 2003), as shown in Figure 5.3.

When people are outraged but the actual hazard is low, the appropriate communication strategy is outrage management. Its goal is to reduce outrage so people don't take unnecessary precautions. The opposite situation—when the danger is high but the public is not very concerned—is precaution advocacy. Its goal is to increase concern for a real hazard in order to motivate people to take preventive action.

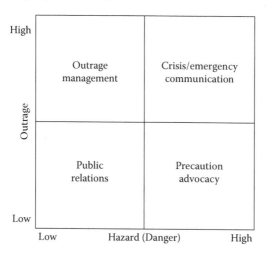

*Figure 5.3* Four different types of risk communication strategy. (From Sandman, P.M. and J. Lanard. 2003. Fear of fear: The role of fear in preparedness...and why it terrifies officials. Peter M. Sandman Risk Communication Website. http://www.psandman.com/col/fear.htm)

When both the outrage and danger are high, crisis communication is in order. It acknowledges the hazard, validates the concerns of the public, and gives people effective ways to act to manage their risk. Situations of low hazard and low outrage are well served by ordinary public relations communications. These communications are brief messages that reinforce whatever appeals are most likely to predispose the audience toward your goals.

These different situations and their associated strategies give rise to an obvious need to understand the perceptions of the public. Risk professionals who do not realize that the public perceives risks differently than they do are in danger of choosing an ineffective risk communication strategy.

### 5.4.1.2 Risk perceptions

What scares people the most? What kinds of conditions increase stress and anxiety? The public takes a rather complex array of factors into account when they form their perception of a risk. The correlation between hazard or actual danger and the public's outrage is not always as high as we might like. Psychometric research has done a great deal to help explain this disconnect.

In the 1980s, Slovic published seminal research in the perception of risk that helped explain people's extreme aversion to some risks and their indifference to others. Fifteen risk characteristics were identified, but many of them proved to be highly correlated to one another, so they were consolidated via factor analysis into two factors called "dread risk" and "unknown risk" (Slovic, 1987; Slovic et al., 1980). As the names suggest, characteristics describing the extent to which the consequences of a risk are dreadful comprise one factor, while characteristics capturing the unknown nature of a risk comprise the other.

Slovic's (1987) research showed that the dread and unknown factors increased or decreased for risks with the characteristics in Table 5.1. Furthermore, research at the time suggested that risks with a high unknown factor were perceived as riskier. Figure 5.4 shows a mapping of the cognitive perceptions of Slovic's subjects. Although it is not a universal mapping, it does provide some insight into the nature of risk perception when combined with the information in Table 5.1.

Since that groundbreaking research, a number of other outrage factors have been found to affect both the perception and acceptability of risks. Some of them are effects on children, the manifestation of effects, trust in institutions, media attention, accident history, benefits associated with the risk, reversibility of effects, origin (natural risks are more acceptable than human-made risks), memorability, moral relevance, and the responsiveness of the risk management process. The riskier a situation "feels" based on these kinds of characteristics, the less acceptable or the more unacceptable it is in people's perceptions.

**Table 5.1** Factors that increase or decrease dread and unknown aspects of risk consequences

| Increases dread | Decreases dread |
|---|---|
| Uncontrollable | Controllable |
| Dread | No dread |
| Global catastrophic | Not global catastrophic |
| Fatal consequences | Nonfatal consequences |
| Not equitable | Equitable |
| Catastrophic | Individual |
| High risk to future generations | Low risk to future generations |
| Not easily reduced | Easily reduced |
| Risk increasing | Risk decreasing |
| Involuntary | Voluntary |
| **Increases unknown** | **Decreases unknown** |
| Not observable | Observable |
| Unknown to those exposed | Known to those exposed |
| Delayed effect | Immediate effect |
| New risk | Old risk |
| Risk unknown to science | Risk known to science |

*Source:*  Slovic, P. 1987. *Science* 236 (4799): 280–285.

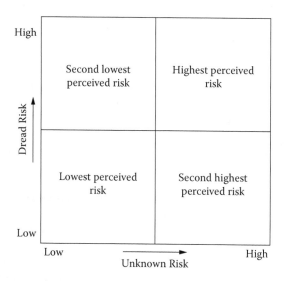

*Figure 5.4* The effect of dread and the unknown on risk perceptions.

### 5.4.1.3   Know and engage your audience

"Audience" is a tricky word; it suggests a one-way communication in its common usage. Here, it is used to identify a particular group of the public that will be the target of a risk communication activity. I will use "public" to mean the collection of all audiences.

There are many different kinds of audiences, and some will be more difficult to persuade or communicate with than others. Take care to avoid the mistake of thinking you have one monolithic audience. Government, industry, academia and research institutions, media, consumers and consumer organizations, and the general public might comprise your audiences. Within the general public are many audience subpopulations that vary based on such things as family situations, locations, education, professions, physical differences, cultural differences, generational differences, language differences, social status, past experience with the risk, prior knowledge of the topic, attitudes toward the responsible organization, belief systems, and so on. Covello and Cohrssen (1989) offered seven rules for engaging the audience that have stood the test of time. They are summarized here to help guide your risk communication efforts.

*5.4.1.3.1   Rule 1: Accept and involve the public as a legitimate partner*   People expect the opportunity to participate in decisions that affect their lives in a democracy. Risk communicators must demonstrate respect for the public; they are going to hold you accountable. Do not attempt to diffuse the public's concern or to preempt any action they may be inclined to take. Instead, aim to develop an involved, interested, reasonable, thoughtful, solution-oriented, and collaborative public-involvement program. Involve people early and in meaningful ways. For example, there may be an important role for the public when preparing the problems-and-opportunities statement, the objectives-and-constraints statement, and the list of questions risk assessment is to answer. If so, that involvement must be planned from the beginning of the risk management activity. This planning is work that would be done as part of the second task in the internal risk communication process (see Figure 5.2).

*5.4.1.3.2   Rule 2: Plan carefully and evaluate your efforts*   You need different communication strategies for different audiences and situations; these strategies must be carefully planned. Begin your communication planning with clear and explicit objectives. Be sure to evaluate your information ahead of time; know its weaknesses as well as its strengths.

Use an effective spokesperson with good presentation and interaction skills. Prepare two or three talking points, word them simply, and learn them cold. Pretest your message whenever it is possible to do so. Pretest with typical people, not activists or community leaders. Always pretest your message before going on television. Then carefully evaluate your efforts and learn from your mistakes.

*5.4.1.3.3    Rule 3: Listen to your audience*    Listen to the audience if you expect them to listen to you. Identify their concerns. They are often more concerned with fairness, trust, credibility, competence, control, caring, and voluntariness than they are with the details of your risk assessment.

Do not assume what people know, think, or want done about the risks. Find out what they are thinking. Never walk into a meeting with no preparation. Use interviews and focus groups to learn. Arrive early to meetings and mingle to find out what people are thinking. Let all interested people be heard. People come to the table with prior life experience, beliefs, personal knowledge, and values. They can be a valuable source of information, especially about social values. Recognize the public's emotions and let them know you have heard them and understand their concerns.

*5.4.1.3.4    Rule 4: Be honest, frank, and open*    Trust and credibility are your most important assets. If you lose them, they are difficult to regain. State your credentials, but do not expect them to validate you. If you do not know the answer to a question, do not fake it. Admit you do not know and get back to them with an answer.

Give people risk information as soon as possible. Do not speculate about or distort the level of risk. Admit mistakes when you make them. Be sure to discuss uncertainties and the strengths and weaknesses of your data. If you must err, err on the side of sharing too much information rather than too little.

*5.4.1.3.5    Rule 5: Coordinate and collaborate with other credible sources*    Avoid conflicts with other credible sources of information. Allies can make the risk communication task easier. Develop relationships with other sources of risk information, preferably in advance of a crisis. Coordinate your messages so the public hears a consistent interpretation of the situation. Determine who is best able to answer questions about risk and let them speak.

Never be blindsided by new information. Monitor the public media on your issue as well as your technical sources. Avoid public disagreements but acknowledge uncertainty when it leads to different interpretations. If others do not coordinate their message with yours, do not argue; be respectful to the other party, but state your position clearly as well as your reasons for it.

*5.4.1.3.6   Rule 6: Meet the needs of the media*   The media are a major channel for disseminating risk information. They are essential to your ability to tell your story and to get information out to your audiences. The media are usually not out to get you; they are out to get a story, so don't be the story. Be accessible to the media and understand their needs for simplicity, conflict, and a "hook" for stories. Supply a hook the media can use. Prepare media materials in advance and tailor them to the specific type of media you use. They should be sufficient for a reporter to tell the whole story in print, video, or audio.

It is wise to establish long-term relationships with media representatives well in advance of a crisis. If a reporter uses you as a reliable source when they need one, they're more likely to come to you when you need to get word out.

*5.4.1.3.7   Rule 7: Speak clearly and with compassion*   Risk assessment is science-based, but communication is not. Avoid technical language, jargon, and acronyms. Use simple, nontechnical language and be sensitive to local norms and expectations about speech and dress. Use concrete, relevant, and simple examples. Vivid metaphors and effective risk comparisons can help to put risks in perspective. People respond better to stories than to theories or a recitation of facts. Tell stories but be consistent with your message.

Be sure to respond to emotions that people express, for example, fear, anger, helplessness, outrage. When responding to emotional outbursts and histrionics, never cut someone off. Speak with them gently. Convey empathy for the person's response while at the same time expressing skepticism over inaccurate things that may have been said. This is not the time to challenge core community attitudes and beliefs!

## SOURCES OF STAKEHOLDER ANGER

Fear
Threat to self
Threat to family
Frustration
Feeling powerless
Feeling disrespected
Feeling ignored

**Source: Risk Communication, Applications, and Case Studies (Neeley, n.d.)**

Never restate a problem in objective terms without the emotional content. Regain control of the discussion by restating the concerns expressed. Watch your body language; it is the greater part of communication.

### 5.4.1.4  Psychographic information

Psychographics is the use of demographics to study and measure attitudes, values, lifestyles, interests, beliefs, and opinions, usually for marketing purposes. Psychographics can also help you deal with your different audiences and to construct messages. For example, some psychographic measures with significance for risk communication are self-esteem, involvement, anxiety, fear, and trust.

Self-esteem embodies our feelings of self-worth and the effectiveness of our own actions. Risks that deal with our health or well-being will be perceived through the lens of our self-esteem. Self-esteem, through its self-efficacy dimension, can affect our perceptions of risk management options like weight loss, exercise, and changes in personal behavior. Groups or individuals with low self-esteem present unique risk communication challenges.

The theory of vested interest (Crano and Burgoon, 2001) identifies four levels of involvement that reflect the degree of concern an audience has regarding a risk. These are:

- Value-relevant involvement
- Outcome-relevant involvement
- Impression-relevant involvement
- Ego-relevant involvement

When people are involved in an issue because it is relevant to their value system, they can be hard to persuade if the situation challenges their values, especially highly engrained ones. To succeed in communication with these groups, your message must reflect their values.

Those involved in an issue because of the personal consequences (i.e., outcome) of the issue can be persuaded if they believe what you propose is in their best interest. The key to the risk communication message is to show them how the topic affects their personal interest and is in their best interest.

Impression-relevant involvement stems from behaviors that serve to create or maintain a specific image of the individual. This self-image tends to inhibit change in general. Effective risk communication must ensure the audience that the actions you want them to take are not silly and that people will not think less of them because they took them.

When a person's involvement is motivated by ego, that person can be difficult to persuade. Messages that threaten the ego evoke defensive reactions, and defensiveness causes people to disparage the source of the message. Consequently, it is important to avoid insulting people.

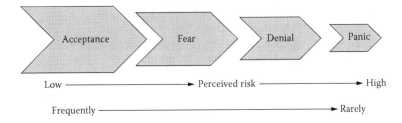

*Figure 5.5* Progression of our reactions to a perceived risk. (From Sandman, P.M. and J. Lanard. 2003. Fear of fear: The role of fear in preparedness…and why it terrifies officials. Peter M. Sandman Risk Communication Website. http://www. psandman.com/col/fear.htm)

When the risk is perceived as high and efficacy is perceived as low, anxiety results. The good news is that anxious people are motivated to seek information. The bad news is that anxiety interferes with our ability to process information.

Fear and trust are adaptive survival processes. Fear rises rapidly and is slow to cease. It is easily reestablished. Trust, on the other hand, is slowly acquired and easily destroyed. Once destroyed, it is very difficult to reestablish.

Sandman and Lanard (2003, 2005) suggest that reactions change with the perception of risk, as shown in Figure 5.5, and that humans usually adapt well to risk. As the perception of the risk increases, our reactions progress from acceptance through fear, denial, and finally panic. Panic, however, is a rare response.

Fear is an adjustment reaction that is natural in a crisis. Sandman and Lanard (2005) say that fear:

- Is automatic
- Comes early
- Is temporary
- Is a small overreaction
- May need guidance
- Serves as a rehearsal
- Reduces later overreaction

Smart risk communicators know this and encourage, legitimize, ally with, and guide these adjustment reactions.

Overreacting to a risk is a natural first reaction when it is new and potentially serious. Typically, we will pause, become hypervigilant, personalize the risk, and take extra precautions that are at worst unnecessary and at best premature.

When this fear grows, it leads to denial, which is less common than fear but more dangerous because it keeps people from taking precautions. Risk communication can reduce denial by legitimizing the fear, taking action by doing something, and empowering people to decide how to respond by providing them with a range of actions they can take.

Panic is a sudden strong feeling of fear that prevents us from reasonable thought or action. Panicky feelings are not unusual, but actual panic is quite rare. We often worry that providing people with unfavorable information or that presenting them with a dire scenario will result in "panic." This can lead communicators to withhold information or to over assure people. The orderly evacuation of the World Trade Center Twin Towers on September 11, 2001, and the January 15, 2009 emergency water landing of a jetliner in the Hudson River, provide vivid examples of how rare panic really is. Most people can cope with and manage their fear. Risk communicators can help mitigate the fear and anxiety by empowering people with information that builds self-efficacy—"This is what you can do..."—and that assures them that response will work. Fearful people need information they can process easily; that means nothing complicated. Keep the message sensitive and simple. Give anxious people specific instructions. Repeat the message as often as possible.

### 5.4.1.5   Risk, stress, and the communication model

Communicating to an emotional and possibly untrusting or, worse, distrustful audience is one of the most difficult tasks you may ever face. Do it well and life may not be simple, but it will be a whole lot easier than if you do it poorly. The basic communication model includes the following components:

- Sender: communicator
- Receiver: public, partners, stakeholders
- Channel: medium used to convey information
- Message: content presented
- Feedback: receiver's response message
- Noise: barriers that may interfere with reception (e.g., physical, receiver's stress level)
- Environment: time and place

During normal risk communications situations when stress is low, trust in the communicator is based on that person's level of competence and expertise. Covello's research (2002) indicates that as much as 85% of trust may be based on these credentials (see Figure 5.6).

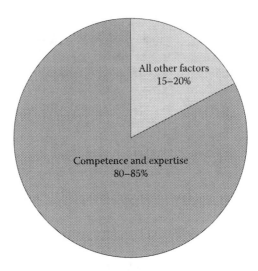

*Figure 5.6* Trust factors in low stress situations. (From Covello, V. 2002. Message mapping, risk and crisis communication. Invited paper presented at the *World Health Organization Conference on Bioterrorism and Risk Communication*, Geneva, Switzerland, http://www.orau.gov/cdcynergy/erc/Content/activeinformation/resources/Covello_message_mapping.pdf)

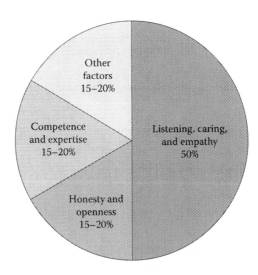

*Figure 5.7* Trust factors in high stress situations. (From Covello, V. 2002. Message mapping, risk and crisis communication. Invited paper presented at the *World Health Organization Conference on Bioterrorism and Risk Communication*, Geneva, Switzerland, http://www.orau.gov/cdcynergy/erc/Content/activeinformation/resources/Covello_message_mapping.pdf)

*Table 5.2* Communication shifts in low- to high-stress situations

| Low stress | High stress |
|---|---|
| Process an average of seven messages | Process an average of three messages |
| Information processed linearly (1, 2, 3) | Information processed in primacy (1, 3, 2) or recency order (3, 2, 1) |
| Information processed at average grade level | Information processed at 4 levels below average grade |
| Focus on competence, expertise, knowledge | Focus on listening, caring, empathy, compassion |

*Source:*   Covello, V. 2002. Message mapping, risk and crisis communication. Invited paper presented at the World Health Organization Conference on Bioterrorism and Risk Communication, Geneva, Switzerland. http://www.orau.gov/cdcynergy/erc/Content/activeinformation/resources/Covello_message_mapping.pdf.

When risks are perceived as high or in crisis situations, communication takes place in high-stress circumstances. Trust factors change rather dramatically during times of high stress, as seen in Figure 5.7. Competence and expertise become far less important, while listening, caring, and empathy become the primary factors for establishing trust. Honesty and openness also appear as important factors. These trust factors are routinely assessed within the first 30 seconds of communication. There is no second chance during stressful circumstances.

The basic communication model changes during high-stress conditions, as summarized in Table 5.2. The effectiveness of the sender now depends on credibility and trust. The receiver's ability to process complex information is reduced, so the messages must be simplified. Feedback is essential to gauging the public's response.

People process information very differently during high-stress situations. We can handle fewer bits of information at a time, and we process it in a different order. Newspapers tend to write for an eighth-grade reading level. If that is the average grade, then during high-stress situations, information is processed at a fourth-grade level.

Mental noise caused by the stress of fear impedes the receiver's ability to accurately process information. To counteract these changes, risk communicators should:

- Simplify the message by lowering the reading level
- Reduce the number of message points to a maximum of three
- Use short sentences
- Use numbers carefully
- Use pictures or graphics to present ideas

**RECOMMENDED TIME LIMITS**

20 minutes combined for all speakers at a public meeting
2 minutes to answer a question at a public meeting
8–10 second soundbites for answering media questions during an
interview
3 minutes for interacting with the public for every minute you
speak

**Source: Eisenberg and Silverberg (2001)**

### 5.4.1.6    *Three M's of risk communication*

Given the potential role of stress in risk communication, there are three categories of tools to consider in risk communication. Referred to as the *three M's of risk communication* (Eisenberg and Silverberg, 2001), they are:

- Message: What to say
- Messenger: Who should say it
- Media: How it should be presented

*5.4.1.6.1   Message*   There can be many different purposes for a risk communication (Fulton and Martinez, n.d.), including:

- Raising awareness
- Educating/informing
- Achieving consensus
- Changing behavior
- Changing perception
- Receiving input

The message needs to be consistent with your purpose.

During the initial stages of message development, there are three helpful questions (Eisenberg and Silverberg, 2001) to consider:

1. What are the three most important things you would like your audience to know?
2. What three things would your audience most like to know?
3. What are the three points your audience is most likely to get wrong unless they are emphasized and explained?

Avoid messages that convey only technical facts. Convey empathy, caring, honesty, openness, dedication, and commitment in your verbal and nonverbal messages. To maximize the information your audience hears, understands, and remembers:

- Structure and organize your message
- Limit your information to three key messages
- Keep your messages short
- Present each message in 7–12 words followed by two to four supporting facts
- Repeat your key messages: Tell them what you are going to tell them; then tell them; and finally tell them what you told them

*5.4.1.6.2  Messenger*   The best spokesperson is not always the topic expert. You need someone who can show empathy, stay organized, understand the audience, and speak clearly—someone with credibility and expertise. Credible speakers have the requisite expertise, but they are also trustworthy and likeable. They are similar to the audience and communicate well nonverbally. Recall that credibility is based on the mix of trust factors identified previously and in the following paragraphs. Expert speakers have advanced knowledge and/or degrees in the area they are speaking about, and they speak with authority, assured in their knowledge. However, the best messenger in a low-stress situation may not be the best messenger in a high-stress situation.

**AVOID**

Humor
Negative terms
Guarantees and absolutes
Complex language
Jargon
Personal beliefs
Attack
Worst case speculation
Numerical details

**Source: Eisenberg and Silverberg (2001)**

People need to know that you care before they will care about what you know. Active listening skills including paraphrasing, providing active feedback, and controlling nonverbal cues are an important part of being perceived as a trustworthy speaker.

To be trustworthy, be balanced. Focus on a specific issue. Pay attention to what the audience already knows and be respectful in tone, recognizing the legitimacy of people's feelings and thoughts. Be honest about the limits of scientific knowledge.

If you make a promise or a commitment, keep it. Come early and stay late. Engage people one on one. Provide a phone number and an e-mail address where you can be reached.

## BODY LANGUAGE

- Make eye contact while slowly sweeping the room
- Avoid darting eyes or staring
- Keep your hands open at about waist level
- Don't cross your arms, make a fist, clasp your hands, put your hands in your pockets, or make large waving hand movements
- Lean slightly forward from the waist
- Avoid slouching and standing or sitting rigidly

**Source: Eisenberg and Silverberg (2001)**

Limit your use of notes and show a high level of organization and logic. Dress professionally; avoid over- or underdressing. Be assertive and avoid hedging. Make sure the audience knows your credentials.

*5.4.1.6.3 Media*   How will you be presenting the information? Media comprise vehicles, channels, and applications for your message appropriate to your audience. Communication vehicles may be written, oral, visual, interactive, computer based, experiential, or technology assisted. Channels include media, advertising, public meetings, one-on-one opportunities, Internet, word of mouth, speaker bureaus, and the like. Examples of applications include such things as fact sheets, pamphlets, reports, news releases, newsletters, web pages, Wiki spaces, public notices, flyers, posters, exhibits, videos, journal articles, fact sheets, tweets, and so on.

Message media are chosen on the basis of impact and influence. Impact refers to how widespread the impact of your message will be, while influence refers to the kind of persuasive influence (e.g., credibility) the channel has. The choice of channel goes back to knowing your audience. Where are they? How do you reach them? Where do they get their information? Do they read newspapers, listen to radio and watch TV, or do they text, tweet, use instant message, e-mail, cruise the Internet, and rely on reference groups for information? Your message must meet them where they are.

### 5.4.1.7 Critical differences in crisis communication

Risk communication has been defined in various ways, but most definitions include some version of a two-way exchange of information and opinion about risks. We have seen previously that when hazard and outrage are both high, we are often engaging in a crisis communication strategy. Glik (2007) defines crisis communication more narrowly as "the exchange of risk-relevant and safety information during an emergency situation." The primary purpose of crisis communication is to motivate the audience to action.

The communication goals are different for more routine risks than for crises. Risk communication addresses what could go wrong and how it could happen. Crisis communication deals with what is happening right now. A crisis is a dynamic, usually unexpected event that involves a significant threat, ongoing uncertainty, and greater intensity than longer-term risk situations (Sellnow et al., 2009). There is not time for many of the best-practice techniques described in the risk communication literature during a crisis. The coordination, collaboration, consensus building, issue resolution, and public-involvement interactions often prescribed will not likely be possible.

---

### CONSEQUENCES OF POOR CRISIS COMMUNICATION

- People may not make good choices or may make them too late.
- Public frustration (or outrage) may develop—once the public reaches an "outrage" state, it is very difficult to go back.
- Messages may be misinterpreted or misunderstood, causing bad feelings.
- Public may start to mistrust the organization.

**Source: Risk Communication, Applications, and Case Studies (Neeley, n.d.)**

---

Whereas risk communication can be planned, tested, and strategic, crisis communication is spontaneous. Risk communication usually takes place before an event occurs, while crisis communication is post event. The risk communication model is multidirectional, proactive, and relatively certain. In a crisis, communication is unidirectional, reactive, and far more equivocal. Seeger and Ulmer (2003) summarize some other potential differences between the two strategies, as shown in Table 5.3.

The person who is a good public relations communicator or even a good risk communicator may not be the best crisis communicator. The outrage can be expected to be greater, but the three M's still apply.

*Table 5.3* Differences between risk communication and crisis communication

| Risk communication | Crisis communication |
| --- | --- |
| Risk-centered: focuses on harm or risk occurring in the future | Event-centered: focuses on a specific event that has occurred and produced harm |
| Messages may include known probabilities of negative consequences and how they may be reduced | Messages address current state or conditions: Magnitude, immediacy, duration, control/remediation, cause, blame, consequences |
| Based on what is currently known | Based on what is known and what is not known |
| Long term (pre-crisis stage) | Short term (crisis stage) |
| Message preparation possible (campaign) | Less preparation (responsive) |
| Personal scope | Community or regional scope |
| Mediated: commercials, ads, brochures, pamphlets | Mediated: press conferences, press releases, speeches, websites |
| Controlled and structured | Spontaneous and reactive |

*Source:* Seeger, M.W. 2002. *Public Relations Review* 28 (4): 329–337.

### 5.4.1.8   Explaining risk to nonexperts

Explaining risk data is not the primary purpose of risk communication, but sometimes it is necessary. Risk assessors have to explain the risk to risk managers. Nonexpert stakeholders and the general public are also going to need scientific and technical information from time to time. There are three principles (Sandman, 1987) for accomplishing this difficult task: simplify, personalize, and use risk comparisons.

*5.4.1.8.1   Simplify*   The challenge is to make hard ideas clear. The best way to do this is to simplify the language rather than the content. You cannot tell the public everything you know, so we need some guidelines for deciding what to say and what to leave out. Sandman and Lanard (2003) suggest three rules of thumb for deciding what gets included and what gets left out.

First, tell people what they need to know. Answer their questions. Provide instructions for coping with a crisis. Stress these things. Second, tell people what they have to know to both understand and feel that they understand the information they are given. The trick here is to know what the audience might get wrong and provide the information that prevents that error. Testing messages is especially useful in this task.

Third, help people understand that there is more than what you are telling them so that additional information at a later date won't make them feel misled. You are building a framework to support an evolving understanding of the problem.

Explaining risk is difficult because people prefer hearing about things that are safe or dangerous. The public is more comfortable with these extremes. To avoid them, risk trade-offs and risk comparisons may be useful.

Although the nature of the risk may, itself, be complex and uncertain, people can understand risk trade-offs, risk comparisons, and risk probabilities when they are carefully explained. Because of the way risk is perceived, the public can be expected to be resistant to the idea that their risk is modest when they are outraged or that it is substantial when they are not. In the long run, effective risk communication relies more on effective ways of addressing the anger, fear, powerlessness, optimism, and overconfidence of the public than it does on finding clever ways to simplify complex information.

The risk information you do prepare is most likely to reach the public through the mass media. Consequently, you are often simplifying risk information for journalists. Journalists are going to simplify the information for their readers. You are more likely to get a better result if you simplify complex information for them than you will if you give them the complex information to simplify. This is especially true for broadcast media that rely on short sound bites.

The greater concern then becomes to avoid oversimplifying the information and misleading the audience. Both your integrity and the public's trust are at stake. The key is to be prepared in advance of this communication with mass media. Know precisely what it is you want the journalist and their audience to take away from your message. In a crisis, you may have little time to prepare, but take the time you have and use it to prepare. If a journalist takes a different approach to the story, you can then quickly answer the less relevant question and follow with the longer prepared answer to the question that "should" have been asked. Alternatively, you are prepared to suggest a focus for the story or interview.

Make fact sheets part of your preparation. This can clarify your most important points without oversimplification. The greatest challenge is when reporters are demanding more information than you have and everyone is hurrying to respond to the crisis. In that case, be honest and warn reporters that you are in a rush and qualify your remarks by acknowledging that you are simplifying the response; then provide an overview of the sorts of information you lack or are omitting for the sake of simplification.

Think about the things people are most likely to get wrong about your message and then provide information to prevent this mistake or discuss the mistake directly. As you and the public find out more about the situation, you want to make sure your simplification holds up as solid and accurate rather than as misleading. There is nothing wrong with being incomplete. Being incorrect is another matter.

*5.4.1.8.2 Personalize*   Make it personal, and the public is much more likely to understand the risk. Experts tend to gravitate toward the big (societal) picture and policy issues, while the audience for your risk information is interested in the smaller (personal) picture and their own options. Individual voluntary decisions are very different from social policy decisions. Ordering the city of Galveston, Texas, to evacuate is a fundamentally different kind of decision than deciding that you want to leave the island. You may be more concerned about the societal risk, but you should be prepared to talk about both.

---

**PERSONALIZE**

"Persons not heeding evacuation orders in single family, one or two-story homes will face certain death."

**National Weather Service, Hurricane Ike warning for Galveston, September, 2008**

"The best way to guard against the flu is to get vaccinated, which helps to protect you, your loved ones, and your community."

**CDC official, seasonal flu vaccination, September, 2006**

---

It helps to understand the reporter's or the audience's viewpoint. Personalizing the issue brings it to life. It makes the abstract concrete. A focus on real people making real decisions is the best way to personalize a risk. The personal judgments of the experts are often a powerful indicator for the public.

Sometimes, the scientist must go against their instinct for the sake of good risk communication. Science is devoted to abstraction and deriving principles and theories from data. The public, on the other hand, wants concrete, specific, and personal information, especially when it comes to novel risks. Examples, anecdotes, and images help to personalize a risk.

Compare a leaking landfill to coffee grounds, a flood to a bathtub overflow, finding the source of a food-borne disease outbreak to finding a needle in a haystack. Good communication relies on vivid and memorable examples and images.

*5.4.1.8.3 Risk comparisons* Risk comparisons are controversial. Some experts like to avoid them; others embrace them as a useful tool for explaining risk to nonexperts. The alternative—providing the risk estimate details—is often not practical. In general, the public does not understand the scale or the units of measurement. What is $7 \times 10^{-7}$? Who knows what a picocurie is or what CFS or CFU mean? For that matter, who knows if a milliliter is a little or a lot? Worse, the consequences and endpoints are often intimidating, threatening, or unattractive. Flesh-eating bacteria, increased lifetime risk of cancer, lost life expectancy, disease, habitat destruction, and so on, are hard to understand and unpleasant to contemplate.

### RISK COMPARISONS CAN HELP WHEN...

1. The source of the comparison has high-credibility and is more or less neutral.
2. The situation is not heavily laden with emotion.
3. The comparison includes some acknowledgment that factors other than relative risk are relevant, that is, the comparison does not dispose of the issue.
4. The comparison aims at clarifying the issue, not at minimizing or dismissing it.

**Source: Covello et al. (1988)**

The challenge is to find a middle ground between safe and dangerous and to present scientific facts that are comprehensible to the audience. Risk comparisons are an option. They help make risk numbers more meaningful and put risks into perspective by comparing this risk to other risks. Covello et al. (1988) have developed a taxonomy of risk comparisons that provides a useful guide to this option:

- The most acceptable risk comparisons are:
  - Comparisons of the same risk at two different times
  - Comparisons with a standard
  - Comparisons with different estimates of the same risk

- Less desirable risk comparisons are:
  - Comparisons of the risk of doing something versus not doing it
  - Comparisons of alternative solutions to the same problem
  - Comparisons with the same risk as experienced in other places
- Even less desirable risk comparisons are:
  - Comparisons of average risk with peak risk at a particular time or location
  - Comparisons of the risk from one source of a particular adverse effect with the risk from all sources of that same adverse effect
- Marginally acceptable risk comparisons are:
  - Comparisons of risk with cost, or of one cost/risk ratio with another cost/risk ratio
  - Comparisons of risk with benefit
  - Comparisons of occupational risks with environmental risks
  - Comparisons with other risks from the same source
  - Comparisons with other specific causes of the same disease, illness, or injury
- Rarely acceptable risk comparisons are:
  - Comparisons of two or more completely unrelated risks
  - Comparison of an unfamiliar risk to a familiar risk

Concrete examples of these can be found at http://www.psandman. com/articles/cma-4.htm.

---

**SCALE COMPARISONS**

One-in-a-million: One drop of gasoline in a full-size car's tankful of gas

One-in-a-billion: One four-inch hamburger in a chain of hamburgers circling Earth at the equator two and half times

One-in-a-trillion: One drop of detergent in enough dishwater to fill a string of railroad tank cars 10 miles long

One-in-a-quadrillion: One human hair out of all the hair on all the heads of all the people in the world

**Source: Covello et al. (1988)**

---

Comparisons must be relevant to your audience. Those rarely acceptable risk comparisons often turn out to be false arguments, based on a flawed premise. Risks have certain contextual characteristics for the audience, as we saw in the discussion of risk perceptions. The comparisons should not contradict any of the important risk characteristics. In other words, do not compare a familiar risk to an unfamiliar one or a voluntary risk to an involuntary one, and so on. The risk comparisons must be appropriate and truly comparable in the eyes of the audience. Use them with caution.

### 5.4.1.9   Explaining uncertainty

Sometimes, risk assessors are the risk communicators. There will always be uncertainty in risk assessment. When explaining uncertainty to risk managers, the job falls to the assessors. When explaining uncertainty to the public, professional risk communicators may be involved. In either case, there are a number of simple rules of thumb (Sandman 2010a, 2010c) that will make the task easier.

---

**TWELVE TIPS FOR EXPRESSING UNCERTAINTY**

1. Ride the risk communication seesaw.
2. Try to replicate in your audience your own level of uncertainty.
3. Avoid explicit claims of confidence.
4. Convert expert disagreement into garden-variety uncertainty.
5. Make your content more tentative than your tone.
6. Show your distress at having to be tentative and acknowledge your audience's distress.
7. Explain what you have done or are doing to reduce the uncertainty.
8. Do not equate uncertainty with safety—or with danger.
9. Explain how uncertainty affects precaution-taking.
10. Don't hide behind uncertainty.
11. Expect some criticism for your lack of confidence.
12. Don't go too far.

**Source: Sandman (2004)**

---

Acknowledge uncertainty from the outset. Do not wait for someone else to discover what you do not know. Bound your uncertainty with a range of possibilities that are credible.

Clarify that you are more certain about some things than others. Tell people:

- What you know for sure
- What you think is almost but not quite certain

- What you think is probable
- What you think is a toss-up
- What you think is possible but unlikely
- What you think is almost inconceivable

Tell people what has been done and what you continue or plan to do to reduce the uncertainty. If you are going to be unable to reduce the uncertainty further, say so. Report everyone's estimates of critical uncertain values, not just your own. Never hide behind uncertainty. If the existence of a problem is uncertain but likely, say so. Neither should you perpetuate uncertainty. If there are things you can do to answer the uncertain questions, do them.

No evidence of an effect is not evidence of no effect. Be especially careful not to say there is no evidence of a particular effect if you have not looked for the evidence.

Let people know when finding out for sure is less important than taking appropriate precautions now. Acknowledge that people disagree about how to respond to uncertainty and that different people may do different things: "Based on the information available I have decided I will not get the swine flu shot, but my wife is going to." Help people become involved in reducing uncertainty for themselves. Give them ways to learn about their own vulnerability. Tell them how to learn about their flood risk; let them know how to get up-to-the-minute information about the neighborhoods that may be affected by the spill. Show them how to find the batch number and date on the recalled peanut butter, and so on.

Research shows that acknowledging uncertainty diminishes the perception of your competence while it increases people's judgment of your trustworthiness. Rarely do we say things like:

> "I have no idea if the side effects of the swine flu vaccine are more or less dangerous than the risks of going unvaccinated. Because of the speed with which the vaccine was developed, no one has any data to estimate that yet."
>
> "The source of this latest outbreak of salmonellosis is not yet known; the evidence is mixed and very confusing."

Experts rarely say they do not know something, and they probably should do so far more often. No one likes to sound ignorant, so we often focus on what we do know, inadvertently leaving out important or useful information about what we do not know. Consequently, experts may sound more certain than they really are. If you sound certain and turn out to be wrong, credibility and trust can be grievously wounded. The best way to ensure that the media do not make you sound more certain than you are is to proclaim your uncertainty. Indeed, part of the risk assessor/communicator job is to be more precise about uncertainty and the level of confidence in their results and in what they are saying.

Another human trait is to be biased toward providing too much reassurance. Optimism is one of our fundamental biases. Uncertainty is not symmetrical: We tend to underplay negative outcomes and overplay positive ones.

## 5.4.2 Public involvement

As noted earlier, public/stakeholder involvement is sometimes considered part of risk communication and sometimes seen as a separate process. Its basic purpose is often to increase awareness or to build public support for a course of action. Public involvement is not going to be required for all risk management activities, whereas some amount of risk communication may be. Consequently, we will restrict our consideration of the topic to a brief review of some public-involvement practices.

The reasons for involving the public in a risk management activity vary, as shown in the public-involvement continuum in Figure 5.8 (Creighton, 2005). The extent of the participation process varies with its purpose. Informing the public is far less intensive than is partnering and developing agreements.

Commonly stated goals for a public-involvement program include the following:

- Incorporate public values into decisions
- Improve the substantive quality of decisions
- Resolve conflict among competing interests
- Build trust in institutions
- Educate and inform the public

That the public should have a say in decisions that affect their lives is one of the core values of public involvement. The risk analysis team

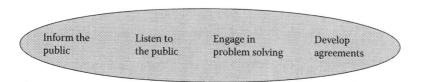

*Figure 5.8* Varying intensity of different public-involvement activities. (From Creighton, J.L. 2005. *The Public participation handbook: Making better decisions through citizen involvement.* San Francisco: Jossey-Bass.)

needs to seek out and involve those potentially affected by the subject risks and their management decisions. In a good public-involvement program, the public's contributions will help define the problems and the risk management objectives. They will have the opportunity to exchange information and opinions and influence decisions. A good public-involvement program communicates how that will happen. The program should convey the interest of the decision makers while it simultaneously meets the process needs of participants. The best programs let participants help define how they will participate.

Involving the public improves the quality of decisions and, through consensus building, it also minimizes cost and delay that can result from processes that exclude the public and leave them no option for participation other than adversarial ones. Public involvement builds trust and helps an organization maintain its credibility and legitimacy. A program that anticipates public concerns and attitudes is easier to implement.

### 5.4.2.1  Planning stakeholder involvement

Creighton (2005) offers a blueprint for developing a public-involvement program, which is summarized in Figure 5.9, where SH stands for stakeholder. The first step is the analysis of the decision context, a subject that was covered in Chapter 3. To adapt this step to include developing a participation program, a few more questions might be added, such as:

- Who needs to be involved in the decision analysis?
- Who is the decision maker?
- What is the decision being made or problem being addressed?
- What are the steps in the decision-making process?
- When will they occur?
- What institutional constraints or special circumstances could influence a stakeholder's participation process?
- Is stakeholder involvement needed?
- If so, what level of participation?
- Will the decision be controversial?
- Will the decision require trade-offs of one value for another?

A good process begins by being clear about why you want public involvement. Do you want a better-informed public? Is it to fulfill legal requirements or to give the public a voice before a decision is made? Do you need support or informed consent? Must you have buy-in for success? Are you trying to change behaviors or save lives?

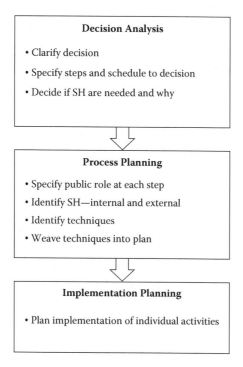

**Figure 5.9** Blueprint for developing a public involvement program. (From Creighton, J.L. 2005. *The Public participation handbook: Making better decisions through citizen involvement.* San Francisco: Jossey-Bass.)

Planning the participation process can also be guided by some questions:

- Who needs to be on the planning team?
- What are the issues?
- Who are the audiences/publics?
- What is the level of controversy and how do we prepare for it?
- What do we want to accomplish at each step?
- What are our stakeholder-involvement objectives?
- What do stakeholders need to know to participate effectively?
- What do we need to learn from stakeholders?
- Do special circumstances affect our techniques?
- What techniques are best?
- What will we include in the plan?

Identifying stakeholders is especially important to ensure that no one is left out and to reach all parties interested in the issue. It is helpful to consider who benefits or loses in a given situation and who uses the relevant and affected resources. Different people and groups can be expected to participate in your process to varying extents. You need effective techniques to involve them all. Information exchange remains the goal of these activities.

## LEVELS OF PARTICIPATION

1. Unsurprised apathetics—do not participate, have little interest
2. Observers—keep abreast and generally do not participate
3. Commenters—very interested, will attend meeting or send letter
4. Technical reviewers—other agencies, peers
5. Active participants—commit time and energy in order to influence decisions
6. Co-decision makers—those who will make or veto a decision

**Source: Creighton (2005)**

You may need to explain the nature of the risk management activity and the decision process. You may want to know how different groups see the problem, who sees themselves as affected, as well as how the problem affects them. One key to good public involvement is to not let the issue slip from view. Although you cannot expect less active participants to sustain interest over a long time, bear in mind that suspicion often grows when an issue disappears. Use a variety of techniques to keep people productively involved in your process. Participation is especially important in the weeks leading up to decision points, and there may be many decision points in a risk management activity.

Implementing a good participation plan will take a mix of skills. You will need a spokesperson, technical experts, and facilitators. You may also need people with a wide array of communications skills. Do your homework and take care not to surprise elected officials or other community leaders and opinion makers. See to the needs of the media. If you are meeting with the public, visit the site in advance. Be sure to back up your technology, have a Plan B, and never outnumber the public.

There are many effective ways to communicate, and technology is growing the list of possibilities all the time. Even though communication is a two-way process, it is convenient to think of "to" and "from" techniques as seen in Table 5.4.

Although one must remain aware of the digital divide that can separate different audience segments, it is exciting to consider the new possibilities for communication and participation that the Internet provides. Online learning

*Table 5.4* Traditional and Internet to-and-from communication techniques

| Traditional to | Internet to | Traditional from | Internet from |
|---|---|---|---|
| Briefings | Data, models, reports | Advisory group or task force | Web conferencing |
| Exhibits and displays | Twitter | Charette | Wiki spaces |
| Feature stories | Hotline | Coffee klatch | Virtual communication |
| Repositories | Up-to-the-minute information | Computer simulation | Interactive websites |
| Mailings | Chatroom, discussion boards | Consensus simulation | Interactive websites |
| Media interviews | Multimedia | Field trip | Shared spaces Blogs Photo sharing |
| Media kits | Interactive | Focus groups | |
| Talk shows | Downloads | Hotlines | |
| News conferences | Distance learning | Interviews | |
| Newsletters | Published information about events | MCDA | |
| News releases | Podcasts | Shared vision planning | |
| Newspaper inserts and advertisements | Instant messaging Blogs Photo sharing | Large groups/ small group meetings | |
| Panels | | | |
| Presentations | | | |
| PSAs | | | |
| Symposia | | | |

classrooms, real-time chat, Twitter, instant messaging, podcasts, Wiki spaces, collaborative working environments, web conferencing, YouTube videos, Instagram, Facebook, interactive learning tools, data visualization techniques, Google, and all manner of emerging social networking techniques and tools make this an exciting time to be interested and active in public involvement.

The way people are working is changing. More and more collaborative work environments are popping up. More and more work is becoming defined by Tapscott and Williams' (2006) four organizing principles:

- Open: all are welcome
- Peered: no one is in charge

- Shared: communal ownership
- Global: worldwide

Now is a great time to use technology to experiment, innovate, and collaborate. Imagine asking the world to help you solve your problem—and getting an answer! Think about using technology so that affected citizens can participate in a more active way. Spread your wings and fly, experiment with new technologies, and vary your approach.

## 5.4.3   Conflict resolution

There will be times when external risk communication includes public involvement, and some public involvement may require conflict resolution. Conflict resolution or consensus communication is often used to bring a number of parties to consensus on how to manage a risk. It is an effort to get people on "the same page." It is most useful for addressing particularly contentious, controversial, or divisive issues (Neeley, n.d.). Although there are many reasons for conflict, three are almost inevitable (Deep and Sussman, 1997) in a risk management activity. Ours is a world of increasing complexity and rapid change. A consequence of that is growing diversity. Three television networks once exhausted the broadcast options for the United States. The amount of options now numbers in the hundreds, and each of these options has viewers in the many thousands or even millions. The first inevitability is that different people want different things. There are few risk management solutions that will satisfy everyone.

---

### PRINCIPLES OF CONSENSUS COMMUNICATION

- Ensure stakeholder or audience participation early and throughout the risk analysis process.
- Listen to and honestly address the public's specific concerns.
- Convey the same information to all segments of your audience.
- When possible, allow stakeholders to participate in risk management decisions.
- Ensure there are effective feedback mechanisms between the communicators and stakeholders.
- Plan how you will balance the interests of various stakeholders.
- Address uncertainty.

**Source: Neeley (n.d.)**

---

Second, risk management activities involve and affect people. To affect people is inevitably to experience conflict. People will miscommunicate, misunderstand, jump to conclusions, suffer bruised egos, hold incompatible beliefs, and have incompatible needs. Humanity breeds conflict.

Third, limited resources mean even the winners in decision processes rarely get exactly what they want. Instead, we are often "satisficing," that is, trying to get the best situation possible given the available options and constraints. For the losers in a decision process, the situation is more dire, so conflict flares readily. Given the inescapable nature of conflict, conflict management may at times be one of the risk manager's most needed skills and one of risk communication's critical tasks.

Deep and Sussman (1997) offer a treasure trove of practical lists for managing conflict productively. Eleven different lists comprising 105 different ideas are included in their conflict management chapter. It is a great place for the novice to begin. There is also a rich professional literature on conflict management (see, for example, Burton, 1968; Kelman and Fisher, 2003; Kriesberg, 1998), and three forms of conflict management are addressed in the literature. These are conflict settlement, conflict resolution, and conflict transformation. Conflict settlement includes any conflict strategy that aims at a definite end of the conflict without necessarily addressing its basic causes (Reimann, 2004). Conflict-resolution approaches include strategies that can be used to find an exit from the conflict's damaging dynamic that aim at reaching a satisfactory solution for all parties involved. Galtung (2000), Lederach (1995), and others have suggested that the conflict context, its structure, the parties involved, and the general conflict issues may at times be transformed into a more agreeable situation.

Like the topic of public involvement, conflict resolution is too complex and too well developed elsewhere to address it in detail here. It is, however, important to understand that conflict resolution may be considered part of the risk communication program in the broadest constructions of the risk communication component.

## 5.5   Summary and look forward

Risk communication has both internal and external tasks. Internally, the coordination between risk managers and assessors is essential to the success of the risk analysis process. Not too many years ago, many thought managers and assessors may need to be separated almost to the point of sequestering the assessors so their objective work would not be tarnished by the subjective concerns of managers. Now we know better and recognize the importance of collaboration, coordination, and cooperation between managers and assessors.

The external communication task usually receives most of the emphasis in discussions of risk communication, and the extent of this task varies from one context to another. The narrower view of the risk communication component focuses on specific risk and crisis communications. An increasingly more common, broader view of this component includes those communications, but may also include public-involvement and conflict-resolution responsibilities.

The hazard and outrage dimensions of risk necessitate at least four types of risk communication strategies. These dimensions can affect the perception of risk, which is an important consideration for both risk managers and risk communicators. There are many unique challenges to effective risk communication, not the least of which is understanding the special challenges of communicating with people who are stressed and fearful. The three M's of risk communication—message, messenger, and media—are an important focus for any risk communication process.

Because the risk analysis process is for making decisions under uncertainty, risk communicators must develop skill at explaining risk and critical uncertainties to nonexperts. This is a task that is aided by simplifying, personalizing, and using risk comparisons. Learning to express uncertainty effectively and developing more effective techniques for communicating complex scientific information and its attendant uncertainty remains a challenge for all risk communicators.

With the three risk analysis components now described, let us once again draw a sharp distinction between the risk analysis sciences, as characterized by these three tasks, and the actual practice of the risk analysis sciences. The private sector has been increasingly, and in some instances aggressively, adopting and practicing enterprise risk management as a strategic and operational framework. Enterprise risk management uses risk management as the overarching concept that includes the three tasks, risk management, risk assessment, and risk communication. As long as you draw a distinction between the science and the practice of risk analysis, the language is a little less confusing. Chapter 6 presents an overview of the enterprise risk management process.

## References

Burton, J.W. 1968. *Systems, states, diplomacy and rules.* Cambridge, U.K.: Cambridge University Press.

Chess, C., and B.J. Hance. 1994. *Communicating with the public: Ten questions environmental managers should ask.* New Brunswick, NJ: Center for Environmental Communication.

Chess, C., B.J. Hance, and P.M. Sandman. 1989. *Planning dialogue with communities: A risk communication workbook.* New Brunswick, NJ: Rutgers University, Cook College, Environmental Communication Research Program.

Covello, V. 2002. Message mapping, risk and crisis communication. Invited paper presented at the *World Health Organization Conference on Bioterrorism and Risk Communication*, Geneva, Switzerland. http://www.orau.gov/cdcynergy/erc/Content/activeinformation/resources/Covello_message_mapping.pdf.

Covello, V.T., and F.H. Allen. 1988. *Seven cardinal rules of risk communication*. OPA-87-020. Washington, DC: Environmental Protection Agency.

Covello, V.T., and J.J. Cohrssen. 1989. *Risk analysis: A guide to principles and methods for analyzing health and environmental risks*. Washington, DC: Council on Environmental Quality.

Covello, V.T., D.B. McCallum, and M. Pavlova. 1989. Principles and guidelines for improving risk communication. In Covello, V.T., D.B. McCallum, and M. Pavlova (eds.), *Effective risk communication: The role and responsibility of government and non-government organizations*, pp. 3–19. New York: Plenum Press.

Covello, V.T., and M.W. Merkhofer. 1993. *Risk assessment methods: Approaches for assessing health and environmental risks*. New York: Plenum Press.

Covello, V.T., and J. Mumpower. 1985. Risk analysis and risk management: An historical perspective. *Risk Analysis* 5 (2): 103–120.

Covello, V.T., R. Peters, J. Wojtecki, and R. Hyde. 2001. Risk communication, the West Nile Virus epidemic, and bioterrorism: Responding to the communication challenges posed by the intentional or unintentional release of a pathogen in an urban setting. *Journal of Urban Health* 78 (2): 382–391.

Covello, V.T., and P.M. Sandman. 2001. Risk communication: Evolution and revolution. In Wolbarst, A.B. (ed.), *Solutions to an environment in peril*, pp. 164–178. Baltimore, MD: Johns Hopkins University Press.

Covello, V.T., P.M. Sandman, and P. Slovic. 1988. *Risk communication, risk statistics, and risk comparisons: A manual for plant managers*. Washington, DC: Chemical Manufacturers Association.

Crano, W.D., and M. Burgoon. 2001. Vested interest theory and AIDS: Self-interest, social influence, and disease prevention. In Butera, F. and G. Mugny (eds.), *Social influence in social reality: Promoting individual and social change*, pp. 277–289. Seattle, WA: Hogrefe & Huber.

Creighton, J.L. 2005. *The Public participation handbook: Making better decisions through citizen involvement*. San Francisco: Jossey-Bass.

Deep, S., and L. Sussman. 1997. *Smart moves: 140 checklists to bring out the best in you and your team*. Rev. ed. Cambridge, MA: Perseus Publishing. http://www.questia.com/library/book/smart-moves-140-checklists-to-bring-out-the-best-in-you-and-your-team-by-sam-deep-lyle-sussman.jsp.

Eisenberg, N.A., and B.R. Silverberg. 2001. *Food safety communication primer: A guide for conveying controversial or sensitive food safety information to concerned audiences*. College Park, MD: Joint Institute for Food Safety and Applied Nutrition.

Fischhoff, B. 1986. Helping the public make health risk decisions. In Covello, V.T., D.B. McCallum, and M. Pavlova (eds.), *Effective risk communication: The role and responsibility of government and non-government organizations*, pp. 111–116. New York: Plenum Press.

Fischhoff, B. 1995. Risk perception and communication unplugged: Twenty years of progress. *Risk Analysis* 15 (2): 137–145.

Fischoff, B., P. Slovic, S. Lichtenstein, S. Read, and B. Combs. 1978. How safe is safe enough? A psychometric study of attitudes towards technological risks and benefits. *Policy Sciences* 9: 127–152.

Food and Agricultural Organization and World Health Organization (FAO/WHO). 2004. United Nations. *Codex Alimentarius Commission, procedural manual.* 14th ed. Rome, Italy: FAO.

Food Insight. 2010. Risk communicator training for food defense preparedness, response and recovery: Trainer's overview. http://www.foodinsight.org/Resources/Detail.aspx?topic=Risk_Communicator_Training_for_Food_Defense_Preparedness_Response_Recovery

Fulton, K., and S. Martinez. n.d. *Risk communication primer: A guide for communicating with any stakeholder on any issue that impacts your mission.* Houston, TX: Fulton Communications.

Galtung, J. 2000. *Conflict transformation by peaceful means (The Transcend Method), participants and trainers manual.* New York: United Nations.

Glik, D. 2007. Risk communication for public health emergencies. *Annual Review of Public Health.* 28: 33–54.

Hance, B.J., C. Chess, and P.M. Sandman. 1990. *Industry risk communication manual.* Boca Raton, FL: CRC Press/Lewis Publishers.

Heath, R.L., and H.D. O'Hair (eds.) 2009. *Handbook of risk and crisis communication.* New York: Routledge.

Johnson, B.B., and V. Covello (eds.) 1987. *The social and cultural construction of risk: Essays on risk selection and perception.* Dordrecht, Netherlands: D. Reidel Publishing.

Kelman, H.C., and R.J. Fisher. 2003. Conflict analysis and resolution. In Sears, D.O., L. Huddy, and R. Jervis (eds.), *Oxford handbook of political psychology,* pp. 315–357. Oxford, U.K.: Oxford University Press.

Kriesberg, L. 1998. *Constructive conflicts. From escalation to resolution.* Lanham, MD: Rowman & Littlefield.

Krimsky, S., and A. Plough. 1988. *Environmental hazards: Communicating risks as a social process.* Dover, MA: Auburn House.

Lederach, J.P. 1995. *Preparing for peace: Conflict transformation across cultures.* Syracuse, NY: Syracuse University Press.

Lundgren, R.E., and A.H. McMakin. 2009. *Risk communication: A handbook for communicating environmental, safety and health risks.* 4th ed. New York: Wiley.

Neeley, A. n.d. Risk communication applications and case studies. Slide presentation for Risk Analysis 101, Raleigh, NC, USDA APHIS PPQ.

Reimann, C. 2004. Assessing the state of the art in conflict transformation. In *Berghof handbook for conflict transformation.* Berghof Research Center for Constructive Conflict Management. http://www.berghof-handbook.net/articles.

Sandman, P.M. 1987. Explaining risk to non-experts: A communications challenge. *Emergency Preparedness Digest* (October–December): 25–29.

Sandman, P.M. 1989. Hazard versus outrage in the public perception of risk. In Covello, V.T., D.B. McCallum, and M. Pavlova (eds.), *Effective risk communication: The role and responsibility of government and non-government organizations,* pp. 45–49. New York: Plenum Press.

Sandman, P.M. 1999. Risk = Hazard + Outrage: Coping with controversy about utility risks. *Engineering News-Record,* October 4.

Sandman, P. 2004. *Acknowledging Uncertainty.* http://www.psandman.com/col/ uncertin.htm.
Sandman, P.M. 2010a. Dealing with uncertainty. Peter M. Sandman Risk Communication Website. http://psandman.com/handouts/sand13.pdf.
Sandman, P.M. 2010b. Four kinds of risk communication. Peter M. Sandman Risk Communication Website. http://www.psandman.com/handouts/ sand17.pdf.
Sandman, P.M. 2010c. Acknowledging uncertainty. Peter M. Sandman Risk Communication Website. http://www.psandman.com/col/uncertin.htm.
Sandman, P.M., and J. Lanard. 2003. Fear of fear: The role of fear in preparedness... and why it terrifies officials. Peter M. Sandman Risk Communication Website. http://www.psandman.com/col/fear.htm.
Sandman, P.M., and J. Lanard. 2005. Adjustment reactions: The teachable moment in crisis communication. Peter M. Sandman Risk Communication Website. http://www.psandman.com/col/teachable.htm.
Seeger, M.W. 2002. Chaos and crisis: Propositions for a general theory of crisis communication. *Public Relations Review* 28 (4): 329–337.
Seeger, M.W., and R.R. Ulmer. 2003. Explaining Enron: Communication and responsible leadership. *Management Communication Quarterly* 17 (1): 58–85.
Sellnow, T.L., R.R. Ulmer, M.W. Seeger, and R. Littlefield. 2009. *Effective risk communication: A message-centered approach.* New York: Springer.
Slovic, P. 1987. Perception of risk. *Science* 236 (4799): 280–285.
Slovic, P., B. Fischoff, and S. Lichenstein. 1980. Facts and fears: Understanding perceived risk. In Schwing, C. and W.A. Albers (eds.), *Societal risk assessment: How safe is enough?* pp. 124–181. New York: Plenum Press.
Slovic, P., N. Krauss, and V.T. Covello. 1990. What should we know about making risk comparisons? *Risk Analysis* 10 (13): 389–392.
Tapscott, D., and A.D. Williams. 2006. *Wikinomics: How mass collaboration changes everything.* New York: Penguin Group.
United Nations (UN). 1998. Food and Agricultural Organization and World Health Organization. *The application of risk communication to food standards and safety matters.* Rome, Italy: FAO.
University of Minnesota. 2006. Terrorism, pandemics, and natural disasters: Food supply chain preparedness, response and recovery. *Symposium Summary,* November 1, 2006. https://ideas.repec.org/s/ags/umfico.html.

## chapter six

# Enterprise risk management

## 6.1 Introduction

The most difficult balance to strike in this text is that between the risk analysis sciences approach presented up to this point and the risk management in practice approach that may be best characterized by enterprise risk management (ERM), the subject of this chapter. The approaches are, I believe, more alike than not but there are significant differences in vocabulary, focus, and application. Risk management is the overarching and organizing concept for ERM; the same three tasks of risk management, risk assessment, and risk communication are all found in the risk management framework. Science is not called out as often or as explicitly in ERM as it is in risk analysis, but ERM still relies on the objective truth. Uncertainty is important to both approaches but it is often subsumed by risk in the world of ERM. Risk assessments are more numerous and regular, as well as usually less complex, in ERM than compared to a public-sector risk assessment used as the basis for a regulation. Risk communication is a component of both approaches but it tends to be more elaborate in the "risk analysis world" than in ERM.

The working vocabulary is different in ERM because it emerged from the insurance, finance, and banking sectors, which have a more limited array of risks than the public sector. ERM uses terms now familiar to you from earlier chapters in different ways. Risk analysis, for example, is a step in risk assessment rather than an overarching term. A risk profile is no longer a summary of what is known about a risk, in ERM it is a description of any set of risks and, thus, it is what is known about the enterprise level risks an organization faces. In addition, ERM brings its own unique set of terms when it speaks of risk appetite, risk tolerance, risk source, and risk criteria. If you approach these differences a bit like you would a foreign language study, you will find many more similarities than differences, because both of these approaches are derived from a common approach to decision making under uncertainty.

The purpose of this chapter is to present an introduction to the world of ERM. It begins by considering what ERM is and by looking briefly at its history. The chapter then presents two of the more popular models used by ERM practitioners followed by a discussion of risk appetite, risk tolerance, and risk profile before concluding with a summary.

## 6.2    *What is enterprise risk management?*

Chapter 1 mentioned the many risk tribes and dialects in existence. Enterprise risk management is a very distinct dialect that first arose in the insurance industry from which it quickly spread to financial firms. Early in the twenty-first century, it has spread rapidly to nonfinancial firms of all types and now is making inroads with many public institutions like universities, school systems, hospitals, and U.S. government agencies. In the pantheon of all things risk, ERM occupies its own hall. It has been distinguished enough by its nature and purpose to earn its own chapter, but it is not so distinguished in practice to be considered outside the risk analysis sciences. The risk analysis methods found in this text would be considered good ERM practice.

> Enterprise risk management (ERM) is defined by the Committee of Sponsoring Organizations (COSO) as "a process, effected by an entity's board of directors, management and other personnel, applied in strategy-setting and across the enterprise, designed to identify potential events that may affect the entity, and manage risk to be within its risk appetite, to provide reasonable assurance regarding the achievement of entity objectives" (COSO, 2004).
>
> ISO 73:2009 in its definition of terms defines risk management as "coordinated activities to direct and control an organization with regard to risk" (ISO, 2018b).

ERM is afflicted by the same misaligned and confusing terminology that plagues all of the risk sciences. Each tribe has a dialect they are loathe to give up. ERM has been described (Protiviti, 2006) as a "best-of-breed" approach to risk management that consists of different techniques that different companies have implemented in different ways. There is no shortage of risk management standards or ERM models in practice and so there is no shortage of confusion about specialized ERM terms like risk appetite, risk tolerance, and such. Two of the most popular risk management models are the Committee of Sponsoring Organizations (COSO) of the Treadway Commission and International Organization for Standardization (ISO, 2018a) 31000 models, both are summarized later in this chapter. Although both are leaders in the field of ERM, the ISO 31000 model avoids the use of the term enterprise risk management and it eschews the use of other common ERM terms like risk appetite and risk tolerance.

ERM arises from a distinct business orientation and it adopts a more business-oriented spin to its language that includes such terms as risk capacity, risk appetite, risk tolerance, risk metrics, and risk portfolio, for a few examples. This alone distinguishes it from other risk management models.

Most businesses have mission and vision statements supported by a strategic plan that expresses strategic objectives for the organization. ERM is assumed to align with the strategic objectives of the entity. This requires the buy-in of the Board of Trustees and other top-level management of the organization, another distinguishing characteristic of ERM.

The diversity of business objectives guarantees a diversity of alignments of ERM frameworks well beyond what is found among public sector organizations. The value sets applied to risk management decision making also tend to be more pecuniary for ERM than for other risk management models. ERM takes great pains to assure that organizations consider opportunities as well as risks, so risk taking is more commonly a risk management responsibility than in the public sector. Risk assessment is sometimes practiced primarily at the enterprise level through the preparation of a risk profile and it is not nearly as complex or involved as many public-sector risk assessments. Issues and debates about unacceptable, tolerable, and acceptable risks are replaced by risk appetites, tolerances, and management of the entity's portfolio of risks.

A singular accomplishment of ERM has been to encourage firms to put aside their traditional "silo" approach to risk management that compartmentalized and isolated the management of risk. In its place, ERM offers portfolio risk management, a unified, holistic structure that assesses and prioritizes risk in order to manage them in an efficient and more effective manner (Barton and MacArthur, 2015). For example, financial risks would no longer be managed in isolation from marketing, production, reputation, or operations risk. The tendency to overmanage some risks while undermanaging other risks would be eliminated by enterprise-wide risk appetites and tolerances.

There is little, if any, substantive difference in the practice of risk management between the generic model presented earlier and ERM. The devil, in this circumstance, is in how one interprets substantive. The language is different, the model's components have different names, acceptable and unacceptable risks are handled differently, but at the task level, at the thinking level, at the doing level, the two approaches to risk management are not significantly different.

So, think of ERM as the international private sector's adaptation of risk management to fit the needs of for-profit business firms. That system has proven robust enough to also be adaptable to the needs of not-for-profit organizations.

## 6.3   History

ERM is a relatively new development in the relatively young field of risk analysis/risk management. As risk analysis with risk assessment and risk

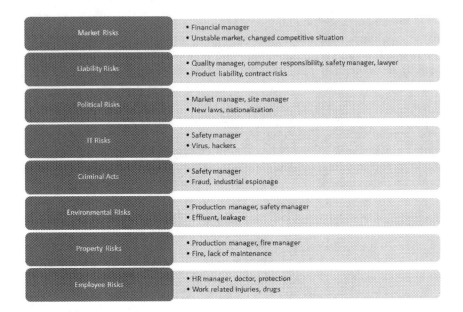

| | |
|---|---|
| Market Risks | • Financial manager<br>• Unstable market, changed competitive situation |
| Liability Risks | • Quality manager, computer responsibility, safety manager, lawyer<br>• Product liability, contract risks |
| Political Risks | • Market manager, site manager<br>• New laws, nationalization |
| IT Risks | • Safety manager<br>• Virus, hackers |
| Criminal Acts | • Safety manager<br>• Fraud, industrial espionage |
| Environmental Risks | • Production manager, safety manager<br>• Effluent, leakage |
| Property Risks | • Production manager, fire manager<br>• Fire, lack of maintenance |
| Employee Risks | • HR manager, doctor, protection<br>• Work related injuries, drugs |

*Figure 6.1* Summary of Gustav Hamilton's risk management circle.

management were being adopted and adapted as a decision framework for public sector regulatory and other decisions, private industry was also expressing interest in risk management. The insurance industry was possibly the first private industry to vigorously embrace ERM and, by the 1990s, financial and banking sector firms were equally immersed in the fledgling practice of ERM. Gradually, more nonfinancial firms took up the practice and today, ERM is widely practiced by a broad array of private industry. A brief timeline for the development of ERM is provided in the paragraphs that follow. Kloman's (2010) work provides the basis for the history prior to about 2000.

In 1955, Dr. Wayne Snider, University of Pennsylvania, suggested "the professional insurance manager should be a risk manager" to Dr. Herbert Denenberg, a colleague. A year later, in 1956, the Harvard Business Review published Russell Gallagher's article, "Risk Management: A New Phase of Cost Control." By 1966, the Insurance Institute of America had developed three examinations leading to the designation "Associate in Risk Management." This corporate insurance management designation broadened the risk management concept.

Gustav Hamilton, a risk manager for Sweden's Statsforetag, developed his "risk management circle" in 1974. His circle, summarized in Figure 6.1[*],

---

[*] Permission to present the circle could not be obtained but images of the circle are readily available on the Internet.

may mark the first attempt to show the interaction of all the elements of the risk management process. The circle presented risks outside of production as dynamic risks (the top three risks in the figure) while risks inside of production or operational risks comprise the remaining risks. Hamilton recognized the wide variety of people who own the risks and must function as risk managers (the top line of each rectangle) as well as recognizing the wide array of risks in each category (the bottom line offers examples). One year later, and two decades after Snider and Denenberg began their discussions, the American Society of Insurance Management changed its name to the Risk and Insurance Management Society (RIMS). That same year, *Fortune* magazine published "The Risk Management Revolution," which suggested the need for coordination of risk management functions within an organization and board responsibility for organizational policy and oversight.

The Committee of Sponsoring Organizations of the Treadway Commission (COSO) was established in 1985 by five private organizations in the United States, as a joint initiative to combat corporate fraud. In 1986, the Institute for Risk Management in London began a program of continuing education that looked at risk management in all its aspects. A series of international examinations led to the designation "Fellow of the Institute of Risk Management." Six years later, the Cadbury Committee issued a report suggesting that governing boards are responsible for risk management in the United Kingdom. That same year, GE Capital used the title "Chief Risk Officer" to describe an organizational function to manage all aspects of risk. Charles Sanford's 1994 paper entitled "The Risk Management Revolution," almost 20 years after the original paper by that name, argued that risk management was a keystone for managing financial institutions. Financial institutions follow a business model that relies on aggregating and disaggregating risk. They have been the cradle of modern ERM since the late 1980s (Pergler, 2012).

Government regulators provided a strong impetus for ERM. During the 1990s, several national standards began advocating that businesses should manage all risks as a portfolio across the enterprise. The first risk management standard, AS/NZS 4360:1995 appeared. This 1995 product of Australia and New Zealand was followed by similar efforts in Canada, Japan, and the United Kingdom. The standard has been revised several times since. In 1996, the Global Association of Risk Professionals (GARP) was established. It provides a global certification program for credit, currency, interest rate, and investment risk managers. In 2003, the Casualty Actuarial Society (CAS) defined ERM as the discipline by which an organization in any industry assesses, controls, exploits, finances, and monitors risks from all sources for the purpose of increasing the organization's short- and long-term value to its stakeholders.

COSO published its "Enterprise Risk Management-Integrated Framework" in 2004. In 2005, the International Organization for Standardization (ISO) undertook an effort to write a new global guideline for the definition and practice of risk management internationally. That guideline "Risk Management-Principles and Guidelines" was completed and released in 2009. It was updated in 2018. The RIMS Risk Maturity Model of 2006 is an online assessment tool recognized as a best practice ERM framework by several national organizations. In 2016, the U.S. Office of Management and Budget Circular No. A-123, *Management's Responsibility for Enterprise Risk Management and Internal Control*, established the requirement for U.S. government agencies to implement an ERM capability in order to improve mission delivery, reduce costs, and focus corrective actions towards key risks. That same year, the Government Accountability Office (2016) published an ERM study on good risk management practices in government.

ERM is still evolving. Looking back, its drivers have been (Fraser and Simkins, 2010):

- Increasing consciousness that a more holistic approach to managing risk makes good business sense
- Studies by effective and authoritative groups that both promote ERM and demonstrate ways to implement and practice it
- Major legal developments which have placed greater responsibility on the board of directors to understand and manage an organization's risk
- ERM's ability to increase firm value

## 6.4    Trends in ERM

This section reviews the contents of several risk management surveys in order to provide a current review of the state of ERM. All of the surveys cited are available online to download.

### 6.4.1    Global business risks

The history of ERM tells part of the story about why interest in risk management has soared in the private sector of the economy. The nature of the risks that most concern the private sector tells another part of the story behind the rising interest in risk management. Although the risks of most concern can vary from location to location and from time to time, the annual Allianz *Business Barometer, Top Business Risks* (Allianz, 2018) provides an insightful view of some of the risks of greatest concern to the world's global businesses.

## TOP 10 GLOBAL BUSINESS RISKS

1. Business interruption
2. Cyber incidents
3. Natural catastrophes
4. Market developments
5. Changes in legislation and regulation
6. Fire, explosion
7. New technologies
8. Loss of reputation or brand value
9. Political risk and violence
10. Climate change/increasing volatility of weather

**Source: Allianz Global Corporate and Specialty. 2018.
Allianz Business Barometer, Top Business Risks for 2018.
London**

## TOP 10 RISKS

1. Damage to reputation/brand
2. Economic slowdown/slow recovery
3. Increasing competition
4. Regulatory/legislative changes
5. Cyber crime/hacking/viruses/malicious codes
6. Failure to innovate/meet customer needs
7. Failure to attract or retain top talent
8. Business interruption
9. Political risk/uncertainties
10. Third party liability

**Source: Aon plc. 2017. Global Risk Management Survey
Aon Risk Solutions**

Business interruption (BI), including supply chain disruption, is the number one risk of concern to global businesses. BI can result from property damages resulting from several of the other top business risks (see text box) or from a break in the supply-chain. The losses due to BI can be higher than the cost of physical damages. Cyber incidents were ranked as the most feared BI trigger in the 2018 survey.

In June 2017, the Petya ransomware attack halted production of a vital vaccine and it brought one of the world's busiest smart ports to a standstill.

Businesses worry about the increasing sophistication of cyber-attacks, which now go beyond the compromise of personal data and intellectual property. Cyber-attacks have risen to the number two risk of concern to global businesses and they are already the top concern in many countries.

From August to September of 2017, Hurricanes Harvey, Irma, and Maria caused $215 billion in damages in the United States and the Caribbean, only $92 billion of which was insured. Natural disasters including hurricanes, earthquakes, droughts, wildfires, windstorms, floods, and the like are the risk of third greatest concern to Global businesses. The impact of natural catastrophes goes beyond physical damage to disrupt the dynamics of societal and industrial operations in affected regions and beyond. Natural disasters are presenting daunting challenges to the insurance industry as well as the organizations directly affected by the disasters.

The fourth-rated risk was market developments. The relatively strong economic performance of the world's three economic superpowers (the United States, Europe, and China) relegated market concerns to a lower rank than it experiences when the global economy is sluggish. Heightened political and policy uncertainty is strong enough to assure this risk remains an important concern.

Changes in legislation and regulation come next. The world continues a fragmentation trend with new protectionist measures growing in numbers with fewer global trade agreements and multilateral platforms. These trends are politically driven. Fire and explosion, the next concern, remain the second major cause of loss for businesses overall. The seventh risk is due to the technological advances of the last decade. Every industry has been penetrated by the digitalization of information; the same interconnectivity that fuels growth, cost optimization, and more flexible interconnectedness also poses significant risks of an inability to deliver products or services, cyber-attacks, infrastructure breakdowns, and new liability scenarios.

Brand accounts for almost 25% of a company's value. Risks to reputation due to health and safety incidents, product recalls, and data security breaches have grown exponentially in an age when a crisis can spread across the globe within minutes. When it comes to political risks, businesses are more worried about terrorism. They do not have to be the direct target of a terrorist attack to feel its effects. An attack in the surrounding area may close a business or impact tourism and spending. The final top 10 risk is due to the perception that the frequency and severity of weather events is increasing.

## 6.4.2   *The financial sector*

The financial and banking sectors have been leaders in developing and adopting ERM. Deloitte Touche conducts an annual survey of financial institutions around the world. The tenth survey (Deloitte Touche Tohmatsu Limited, 2018) found that risk management practices continue to gain wider adoption across the finance industry. Boards of directors devote more time and take a more active role in ERM oversight. The existence of a chief risk officer (CRO) is almost universal (92%) and the CRO is reporting directly to the board of directors and the chief executive officer (CEO). ERM programs are no longer novelties, 73% of institutions report having an ERM program. Another 13% said they are currently implementing an ERM program, while another 6% plan to create one in the future. ERM programs have been a focus of regulatory authorities in the United States/Canada (89%) and Europe (81%) and are more common than in Asia Pacific (69%) or Latin America (38%).

Table 6.1 shows the top risk management priorities for financial firms identified in the survey. The rapid growth of ERM has made attracting and retaining risk management professionals a significant challenge to the industry.

A significant majority of survey respondents rated their institutions as extremely or very effective in managing traditional risks of *liquidity* (84%), *underwriting/reserving* (83%), *credit* (83%), *asset and liability* (82%), *investment* (80%), and *market* (79%).

*Table 6.1* Financial industry risk management priorities identified in Deloitte Touche 10th global risk management survey

| Priority | Firms identifying this priority (%) |
| --- | --- |
| Enhancing risk information systems and technology infrastructure | 78 |
| Collaborating between the business units and the risk management function | 74 |
| Enhancing the quality, availability, and timeliness of risk data | 72 |
| Attracting and retaining risk management professionals with required skills | 70 |
| Establishing and embedding the risk culture across the enterprise | 69 |
| Increasing regulatory requirements and expectations | 67 |
| Identifying and managing new and emerging risks | 61 |
| Collaborating between the risk management function and other functions | 58 |
| Attracting and retaining business unit professionals with required risk management skills | 54 |

Risk management programs for these risks are established with proven methodologies and analytics and relevant data are available. Operational risk proves a greater challenge with 51% rating their institutions as extremely or very effective. Newer types of risk are an even greater challenge because regulatory expectations are less well-defined, and methodologies, analytics, and relevant data are not yet available. The progress has been undeniable, but in the years ahead, risk management is likely to face a growing set of challenges.

### 6.4.3   The state of enterprise risk management

A major distinction of ERM is its tenant that opportunity does not exist without risk. Thus, when risk is taken strategically, new opportunities to accelerate organizational performance emerge. Deloitte (2017) surveyed 300 U.S.-based executives at large organizations about their views on risk management as a means of accelerating business performance. Four key insights were gleaned from the survey results.

First, a value-focused approach to risk strategy yields significant benefits. First among these is heightened financial and operational performance of the corporation. The second benefit is the competitive advantage that results because risk managing businesses manage costs better and improve customer relationships. A third category of benefits is enhanced brand and reputation due to improved risk protection and reputational resiliency.

A second insight is that with change comes challenge. Organizations struggle with risk strategy implementation. Even though 88% of respondents recognize value creation as a key goal of their risk strategies, only 40% believe they have been successful in creating value. The persistence of organizational silos was cited as a top risk-related failure that causes organizations to struggle with implementing a value-focused risk strategy.

The third insight is that timing is everything. Organizations must be prepared to react to a changing landscape. Important shifts are expected in the near future that make it imperative for business leaders to react quickly. Cyber security, for example, has risen to the top of the corporate mind. Interestingly, a little over half of the respondents say that cyber risk is both a threat and an opportunity. Building a risk-aware culture and identifying opportunities for loss avoidance are becoming more important, while improving compliance is becoming less of a focus.

The fourth insight concerns the road ahead for smart risk takers. This begins by breaking down the wall between risk management and strategic planning. Risk professionals and business leaders must share ideas. Business must create a culture where risk is everybody's business. Finally, risk leaders should adopt data analytics to measure risk and predict trends.

*Table 6.2* Selected highlights of the RIMS 2017 ERM benchmark survey

| Finding | Percent of respondents agreeing (%) |
|---|---|
| Have fully or partially integrated ERM programs in operation | 73 |
| ERM is being used to inform and influence strategy | 61 |
| Have a risk management department primarily responsible for ERM | 62 |
| Use ISO 31000 as their guide | 25 |
| Use COSO as their guide | 29 |
| Do not follow a particular standard or framework | 20 |
| Do not have risk appetite and risk tolerance statements | 49 |

The RIMS (2017) survey had almost 397 respondents from 14 different industries, thus it is one of the best indicators of the current state of the ERM art in the entire private sector. Table 6.2 presents selected highlights from the survey. A majority of firms responding have an ERM program in place and about three in five of them use it to influence strategy. About three in five organizations have a risk management department responsible for ERM. Better than half of all firms use either the ISO 31000 or the COSO model as their guide to ERM. Another 20% say they are not using a specific model. About half of the responding organizations do not have a risk appetite or risk tolerances.

The top three things executives expect ERM to deliver are:

- Reasonable assurance that major risks are identified
- Minimize operational surprises and reduced losses
- Aligned risk appetite and strategic risk management

Organizations were asked to rate their effectiveness on several ERM activities using a five-point scale where 1 = not effective at all and 5 = highly effective. Table 6.3 shows the results with the average score for all respondents. Significant improvement is noted in all activities over the previous 2013 benchmark.

The top four values respondents gain from their ERM programs are (primary% and secondary%):

- Increasing risk awareness (24% and 42%)
- Avoiding and/or mitigating risk (24% and 33%)

*Table 6.3* Effectiveness of your organization in selected ERM activities

| ERM activity | 2017 effectiveness score (2013 score) |
| --- | --- |
| Taking action on identified important and relevant risks | 3.8 (2.2) |
| Anticipating and managing emerging risks | 3.3 (2.6) |
| Instilling awareness of risk as a decision-making discipline | 3.3 (2.5) |
| Linking risk management with corporate strategy and planning | 3.2 (2.7) |
| Clearly articulating risk appetite and tolerances | 3.1 (2.9) |

*Source:* RIMS, the Risk Management Society. 2017. 2017 Enterprise Risk Management Benchmark Survey, Executive Report.

- Eliminating silos, that is, viewing the entire portfolio of risks (20% and 29%)
- Increasing certainty in meeting strategic and operational objectives (16% and 28%)

Half or more of all organizations identify the following risks as among those that are addressed by their ERM programs, in order of frequency of mention:

- IT risk management
- Compliance
- Business continuity
- Operations/safety
- Strategic planning
- Legal
- Internal audit
- Human resources
- Security

Although ERM has made notable strides in penetrating private industry, the numerous surveys suggest both the need and desire for continued improvement.

## 6.5   *Enterprise risk management for dummies*

This text, to a great extent, describes the risk analysis experience of an organization that possesses stewardship responsibility for some

*Table 6.4* Selected differences between public and private sector organizations

|  | Public sector | Private sector |
|---|---|---|
| Control and ownership of organization | Government | Private individual and corporations |
| Fundamental objectives | Serve people | Make profit |
| Strategic goals | Influenced by outside forces | Set by organization |
| Revenue | Public sources-tax, duty, penalty, fees | Stocks/loans/sales |
| Accountability | To public and political leaders | To ownership |
| Government influence | Full control | Varying degrees of influence |
| Job security | Greater | Lesser |
| Work environment | Some monopoly power | Competitive |

*Source:* Adapted from Surbhi, S. 2015. "Difference between public sector and private sector." *Key Differences.* May 20. https://keydifferences.com/difference-between-public-sector-and-private-sector.html (accessed December 29, 2017).

public trust. This is the arena in which risk analysis began as a formal science-based approach to decision making. These organizations have often had a more open-ended approach to risk management, in the sense that they may have a wider and at times less well-defined purview of responsibility than private organizations, especially "for-profit" private organizations.

There are some fundamental differences between public and private sector organizations (see Table 6.4) and these differences have influenced and differentiated the practice of risk management in these two sectors.

The fundamental objectives of these two kinds of organizations are different. Public sector organizations focus on serving the general public and looking after their changing interests. Private sector organizations can have varied objectives but the profit motive is representative of most organizations. Private organizations answer to stockholders and boards of directors. Public organizations answer to stakeholders and customers. Because of the differing sources of revenue, public sector organizations can survive inefficient operation, while poorly run private sector firms can quickly go out of business. The public sector focuses on public concerns, but they are watched by interest groups and oversight committees. These differences affect the ways organizations in each sector operate.

Private sector managers can hire quickly. Meeting personnel needs in the public sector can take months to years. Likewise, the time frame for firing people differs by sector. Government budget processes are cumbersome, subject to political wiles, and are anything but adaptable. Purchasing processes are also far more burdensome. Private organizations, by contrast, can use their revenue from sales and investments to buy things when they need them. They also have a quicker procurement process.

Public organizations are subject to a different kind of scrutiny due to the public eye they operate under. Leaders of private organizations do not face this level of scrutiny. They are accountable to their boards of directors and shareholders rather than the public.

Private organizations can set their own strategic goals and then focus resources on accomplishing them. Public organizations are buffeted by prevailing political winds. They are regularly challenged to meet legislative mandates, they face more outside forces, and have far more stakeholders who must be accommodated to some extent. Answering to public officials in pursuit of election victories further challenges accountability. The goals of public organizations can turn dramatically and quickly with the results of an election.

As a result of these differences, the approach of these organizations to risk management is somewhat different too. The public sector tends to utilize a process like that described in Chapter 3. Private sector organizations tend to favor ERM, although there are ample exceptions to each case. The differences between these two approaches are more semantic than substantive. But the semantics are important. This section offers a simplified interpretation of the major differences introduced by the ERM approach.

ERM begins with the strategic objectives of the organization. These will often be found in the strategic plan and they describe what success looks like for the organization. A good strategic plan will provide metrics for measuring progress toward the achievement of these objectives. What a strategic plan does not do is identify those risks that can interfere with the achievement of those objectives. Nor does it identify new opportunities for achieving those objectives. ERM does this and it identifies metrics that can be used to manage those risks. These enterprise-level risks are typically managed by the senior leaders of an organization or its board.

The risks identified have to be assessed. This process of assessing enterprise-level risks is sometimes called creating a risk profile, which helps to identify the risks of greatest concern to the organization. Risk managers then establish an organizational risk appetite for these enterprise-level risks. The appetite identifies the amount of risk the organization is comfortable accepting, while they pursue their strategic objectives. Some organizations may establish risk tolerances for these risks. A risk tolerance identifies the point at which a tolerable level of risk becomes unacceptable. It is usually an upper and/or lower bound on the risk appetite. Public organizations usually assess a risk and then must decide if that risk is acceptable, tolerable, or unacceptable. In a private organization, a risk tolerance identifies the specific points at which risk management measures will be implemented.

Each entity will establish some sort of governance structure to undertake this enterprise-level risk management and to establish the policy, process, and procedures necessary to assure that ERM is implemented horizontally and vertically throughout the organization. Risks are managed jointly in a portfolio rather than individually in silos.

Beyond these distinctions and those in the introduction to the chapter, the process is actually quite similar to the process described throughout this book. An examination of the details of any ERM model will reveal different, if not unique, language and detail. There is much more that unites ERM to the generic risk management process presented here than that divides it.

## 6.6   Risk management standards and guidance

A Google search on the title of this section produces over 123 million entries, many of which are actually directly related to the topic. There is no shortage of entries in this "best-of-breed" competition. A standard is an established norm that is usually voluntary in nature. It is generally promulgated by a standard setting organization. By contrast, a regulation is generally mandatory. Guidance includes the presentation of customs, conventions, guidance documents, frameworks, or company products that may be developed outside of a recognized standard-setting body but which becomes generally accepted practice.

From the many standards and guidance candidates, two are chosen for review in this chapter, they are the ISO and the COSO models. The ISO has issued four primary sources of guidance on risk management. They are:

- ISO Guide 73:2009 Risk Management—Vocabulary
- ISO 31000:2009 Risk Management—Principles and Guidelines
- ISO/IEC 31010:2009 Risk Management—Risk Assessment Techniques
- ISO 31000:2018 Risk Management—Guidelines

### SELECTED STANDARDS AND GUIDANCE

RIMS (2011) provided an overview of six standards and guidelines. They are indicative of the dominant examples in ERM and are:

ISO 31000: 2009 Risk Management—Priciples and Guidelines
OCEG "Red Book" 2.0: 2009 GRC Capability Model
BS 31100: 2008 Code of Practice for Risk Management
COSO: 2004 Enterprise Risk Management—Integrated Framework
FERMA: 2002 A Risk Management Standard
SOLVENCY II: 2012 Risk Management for the Insurance Industry

The introduction to ISO Guide 73 notes "that in addition to managing threats to the achievement of their objectives, organizations are increasingly applying risk management processes and developing an integrated approach to risk management in order to improve the management of potential opportunities." Risk is defined as the effect of uncertainty on the objectives of an organization. An effect is a positive or negative deviation from the expected outcome.

Risk management is said to comprise the "coordinated activities to direct and control an organization with regard to risk." A risk management framework is a set of components that provides the foundations and organizational arrangements for designing, implementing, monitoring, reviewing, and continually improving risk management throughout the organization. It is increasingly common for private industry to adopt an ERM model as its risk management framework. These models vary and are based more or less on the ISO risk management principles. The best ones provide for managing risk across the enterprise.

The COSO ERM framework is the second model summarized in this chapter. The primary reference for this framework is *Enterprise Risk Management—Integrated Framework* (2004). The underlying premise of COSO's ERM framework is that every entity exists to provide value for its stakeholders and every entity faces uncertainty. Uncertainty presents both risk of loss and opportunity for gain. This uncertainty affects an enterprise's ability to achieve its objectives. ERM provides a framework for management to effectively deal with uncertainty and its associated risk of loss and gain. COSO defined ERM as, "The culture, capabilities, and practices, integrated with strategy-setting and its execution, that organizations rely on to manage risk in creating, preserving, and realizing value."

## 6.7    ISO 31000:2018 risk management—guidelines

It bears repeating that this international standard never uses the term enterprise risk management, despite its status as one of the world's foremost ERM models. To be faithful to the document, risk management will be used in this discussion. However, if you hear ERM in its place no one will be offended. The substance of the standard is contained in its definition of terms, principles, framework, and process. Figure 6.2 shows the relationship among the principles, framework, and process. Each component is described in a subsequent section. Eight risk-related terms, down from 29 in ISO 31000:2009, are defined in clause 3 of the standard. Many of these definitions have been adopted by other standards and guidance. The discussion that follows paraphrases ISO 31000:2018.

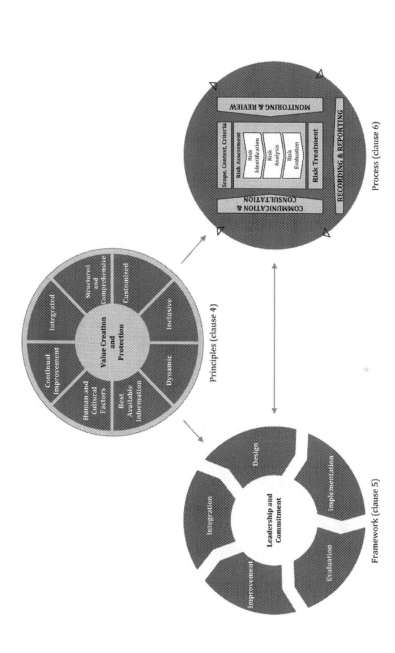

*Figure 6.2* Relationship of the ISO 31000 principles, framework and process. "Copyright ISO. This material is reproduced from ISO 31000:2018 with permission of the American National Standards Institute (ANSI) on behalf of the International Organization for Standardization. The complete standard can be purchased from ANSI at https://webstore.ansi.org. All rights reserved."

## 6.7.1   *ISO 31000:2018 principles*

Below and in Figure 6.3 you will find the ISO principles, which define an effective risk management organization. Risk management is:

- Integrated
- Structured and comprehensive
- Customized
- Inclusive
- Dynamic
- Best available information

These mean that risk management is an integral part of all of an organization's activities. The process is structured and comprehensive in order to produce consistent and comparable results. The framework and process are customized to meet the needs of the organization. It includes appropriate and timely two-way involvement of stakeholders while it enables their knowledge, views, and perceptions to be considered. Risks can emerge, change, or disappear as the organization's external and internal contexts change. The inputs to risk management are based on the best available information and include appropriate consideration of any limitations and uncertainties associated with that information.

**THE ISO PRINCIPLES FROM ISO 31000:2009, STILL INFORMATIVE, ARE THE FOLLOWING:**

- Creates and protects value.
- Is an integral part of all organizational processes.
- Is part of decision making.
- Explicitly addresses uncertainty.
- Is systematic, structured, and timely.
- Is based on the best available information.
- Is tailored.
- Takes human and cultural factors into account.
- Is dynamic, iterative, and responsive to change.
- Facilitates continual improvement of the organization.

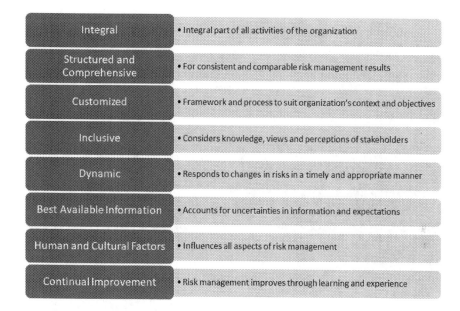

| | |
|---|---|
| Integral | • Integral part of all activities of the organization |
| Structured and Comprehensive | • For consistent and comparable risk management results |
| Customized | • Framework and process to suit organization's context and objectives |
| Inclusive | • Considers knowledge, views and perceptions of stakeholders |
| Dynamic | • Responds to changes in risks in a timely and appropriate manner |
| Best Available Information | • Accounts for uncertainties in information and expectations |
| Human and Cultural Factors | • Influences all aspects of risk management |
| Continual Improvement | • Risk management improves through learning and experience |

*Figure 6.3* ISO 31000:2018 Risk management principles summary. (Adapted from International Organization for Standardization (ISO). 2018a. *ISO 31000:2018 Risk Management Guidelines*. Geneva: ISO.)

## 6.7.2   ISO 31000:2018 framework

ISO describes the risk management framework as the set of components that provides the foundations and organizational arrangements for designing, implementing, monitoring, reviewing, and continually improving risk management throughout the organization. The framework helps to integrate risk management into the organization's activities and functions. Its effectiveness depends on the extent of its integration into the governance of the organization. The ISO framework comprises the elements of Figure 6.4. The specific components of the framework and the way they work together should be customized to the needs of the organization. The organization's risk management leadership and commitment are embodied in the framework.

*Integration.* A strong and sustained commitment by the organization's management is the starting point for risk management. Chief among management's responsibilities are:

- Defining the risk management policy
- Aligning the strategic objectives of the organization with the risk management objectives

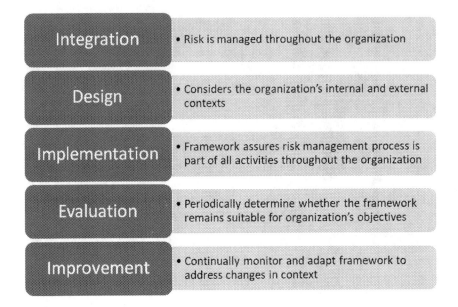

**Figure 6.4** ISO 31000:2018–02 Risk management framework summary. (Adapted from International Organization for Standardization (ISO). 2018a. *ISO 31000:2018 Risk Management Guidelines.* Geneva: ISO.)

- Assigning risk management accountabilities and responsibilities at appropriate levels throughout the organization
- Allocating sufficient resources to risk management
- Ensuring the risk management framework remains appropriate

Establishing the organization's risk management policy is a critical early step. This policy should be communicated appropriately throughout the organization. Management must assure that there is accountability, authority, and appropriate competence for managing risk. This must include identifying risk owners that have both the authority and the accountability to manage risks.

The risk management plan should be integrated into all the organizational practices and processes in a way that it is relevant, effective and efficient. Sufficient resources must be allocated for risk management to assure the necessary people, skills, experience, and competence are available. Training programs must be a sustained integral part of the framework.

Integrating risk management into the activities and functions of an organization requires understanding the organization's governance, structures, and context. Governance guides the course of the organization and management structures translate governance direction into the strategy and objectives required to achieve the organization's desired levels of sustainable performance and long-term viability. Integrating risk management into an organization is a dynamic and iterative process that must be customized to meet the organization's needs and to serve its culture.

*Design.* Management is responsible for the design of the organization's framework for managing risk. This begins by understanding the organization and its context, most importantly the organization's policies and objectives, as well as the strategies put in place to achieve them. When designing the framework for managing risk, the organization should:

• Understand the organization and its context
• Articulate its risk management commitment
• Assign organization roles, responsibilities, authorities, and accountabilities
• Allocate resources
• Establish communication and consultation

*Implementation.* Implementing the risk management framework is obviously one of the critical elements of the framework. Assuring that risk management policy and process are embedded in all organizational processes is a significant and continuous undertaking. Training personnel in the risk management process of the organization is critical to the success of that process. Risk management should be implemented at all relevant levels and functions of the organization as part of its practices and processes. Once it is properly designed and implemented, the risk management framework ensures that the risk management process is a part of all decision-making activities throughout the organization.

*Evaluation.* Monitoring and review of the framework are necessary to ensure that risk management is effectively supporting the organization's performance. Ideally, monitoring will include measuring the organization's risk management performance against indicators. The effectiveness of the framework also needs to be regularly reviewed and modified as warranted.

*Improvement.* The organization should continually monitor and adapt its risk management framework to changes in its external and internal contexts. Based on the results of this monitoring and review, the organization's risk management framework, policy, and plan can be continually improved. The organization should also continually improve the suitability, adequacy, and effectiveness of the risk management framework and the way it is integrated throughout the organization.

### 6.7.3   *ISO 31000:2018 risk management process*

The risk management process describes the manner in which risks are managed. The process can be applied at the strategic, operational, program, or project levels. It is a systematic application of policies, procedures, and practices to the activities of communicating and consulting, establishing the context and assessing, treating, monitoring, reviewing, recording, and reporting risk. This process should be an integral part of decision-making that is integrated into the structure, operations, and processes of the organization.

The ISO risk management process comprises the five steps or stages and three processes seen in Figure 6.5. Some of the sharpest differences from the terminology as used in the majority of this text are encountered here in the ISO risk management process.

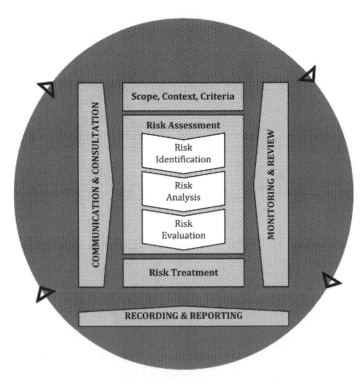

*Figure 6.5* ISO 31000:2018-02 risk management process. (Copyright ISO. This material is reproduced from ISO 31000:2018 with permission of the American National Standards Institute (ANSI) on behalf of the International Organization for Standardization. The complete standard can be purchased from ANSI at https://webstore.ansi.org. All rights reserved.)

The risk management process is applied to a specific risk management activity. This all begins by establishing the scope, context, and criteria that customize the risk management activity. This includes articulating the relevant objectives of the activity. Risk managers will establish the external environment, which may include but is not limited to the organization's social and cultural, political, legal, regulatory, financial, technological, economic, natural, and competitive environment, whether international, national, regional, or local. The internal context of the organization must also be established. The objectives and criteria of a particular project, process, or activity should be considered in the light of the objectives of the organization as a whole. Criteria should reflect the entity's risk appetite and tolerance. The organization should also recognize opportunities to achieve their strategic, project, or business objectives.

The objectives, strategies, scope, and parameters of each individual activity must be established. The ISO description of this particular context is quite extensive and includes identifying and specifying the decisions that have to be made as well as defining the risk assessment methodologies. The primary intent of this stage of the process is to ensure that the risk management approach adopted is appropriate to the circumstances, to the organization, and to the risks affecting the achievement of its objectives.

The ISO defines risk assessment as the overall process of risk identification, risk analysis, and risk evaluation. This differs from this text's definition of risk assessment. The ISO definition includes this text's risk assessment and some of its risk management process.

The ISO's definition of risk analysis is a process to comprehend the nature of risk and to determine the level of risk. This more closely resembles this text's definition of risk assessment.

In the ISO's dialect, risk analysis is a component of risk assessment. In this text's dialect, risk assessment is a component of risk analysis. The language of risk is very messy.

An additional task in this stage is to define appropriate risk criteria for the specific activity. This entails considering how to:

- Measure the nature and types of causes and consequences that can occur
- Define likelihood
- Determine the time frame(s) of the likelihood and/or consequence(s)
- Determine the level of risk
- Ascertain the views of stakeholders

- Establish the level at which risk becomes acceptable or tolerable
- Consider combinations of multiple risks when applicable

The next three stages comprise the risk assessment. It begins with risk identification. The purpose of this stage is to generate a comprehensive list of risks based on those events that might create, enhance, prevent, degrade, accelerate, or delay the achievement of objectives. This should include identifying the risks associated with not pursuing an opportunity. Risk identification is a crucial step because risks not identified will not be analyzed further. Risk identification tools and techniques should be chosen based on what best suits the organization.

The next stage is called risk analysis. This is where an understanding of the risk is developed. In the ISO model, risk analysis provides an input to risk evaluation. It is used to decide whether risks need to be treated, and if so, the most appropriate risk treatment options. ISO's risk analysis is very much like the risk assessment described in Chapter 3. It should consider such things as:

- The likelihood of events and consequences
- The nature and magnitude of consequences
- Complexity and connectivity
- Time-related factors and volatility
- The effectiveness of existing controls
- Sensitivity and confidence levels

Consequences and likelihoods may be expressed qualitatively, semi-quantitatively, or quantitatively depending on the type of risk, the information available, and the intended use of the risk assessment output. Uncertainty should be addressed through a combination of techniques and communicated effectively to decision makers and other stakeholders.

Risk evaluation is ISO's third and final stage in the risk assessment. In risk evaluation, decision makers compare the level of risk determined during the risk analysis process with risk criteria established during the context step. The need for treatment can be determined based on this comparison. Decision making about which risks need treatment and the priority for treatment implementation begins here. All decisions should be made in accordance with legal, regulatory, and other requirements. The purpose of risk evaluation is to support decisions. Risk evaluation can lead to a decision to:

- Do nothing further
- Consider risk treatment options
- Undertake further analysis to better understand the risk

- Maintain existing controls
- Reconsider objectives

Once the assessment is completed, the final stage is risk treatment. Risk treatment is an iterative process of formulating and selecting risk treatment options and implementing one or more options for modifying risks. Risk treatment options include:

- Avoiding the risk by deciding not to start or continue with the activity that gives rise to the risk
- Taking or increasing the risk in order to pursue an opportunity
- Removing the risk source
- Changing the likelihood
- Changing the consequence
- Sharing the risk with another party or parties (including contracts and risk financing)
- Retaining the risk by informed decision

Choosing the best treatment option involves balancing the costs and benefits of implementation. The ISO suggests these decisions should include consideration of risk treatment that is not justifiable on economic grounds. Treatment options can be considered and applied either individually or in combination. The risk treatment must be planned and implemented. Once the treatment has been assessed, a risk treatment plan should be developed to document how the chosen treatment options will be implemented.

The information provided in the treatment plan should include:

- The selection rationale, including the expected benefits
- Identification of those accountable and responsible for approving and implementing the plan
- The proposed actions
- The required resources
- Appropriate performance measures
- Relevant constraints
- Reporting and monitoring requirements
- A schedule for taking and completing actions

The effectiveness of the treatment must be assessed. A risk treatment can introduce risks. One such risk is the failure or ineffectiveness of the risk treatment measures. Treatment can also introduce secondary risks. Both of these classes of risk need to be assessed, treated, monitored, and reviewed. Then it is necessary to decide whether the remaining risk is acceptable and if it is not, the process should be iterated to prescribe further treatment.

The first process is communication and consultation with internal and external stakeholders. Communication should address the risk itself, its causes, its consequences (if known), and the measures being taken to treat it. Consultation provides input and feedback opportunities to support decision making and it suggests that a team approach to risk management will be employed. Plans for communicating and consulting need to be developed at the outset of a risk management activity. Communication and consultation with appropriate external and internal stakeholders should take place within and throughout all steps of the risk management process. Communication and consultation is intended to facilitate truthful, relevant, accurate, and understandable exchanges of information.

The second ongoing process is monitoring and review. Both activities have to be planned and implemented, with responsibilities for monitoring and review clearly defined. These activities are to ensure that risk controls are effective and efficient in both design and operation as well as to assure and improve the quality and effectiveness of the risk management process design, implementation, and outcomes.

The third and final process is recording and reporting. This process is intended to:

- Communicate risk management outcomes and activities across the organization
- Support decision making with information
- Improve risk management activities
- Assist interaction with stakeholders

## 6.8   COSO's enterprise risk management integrated framework

COSO describes ERM as a process that is executed strategically by the people of the enterprise. It is applied horizontally and vertically throughout the organization and it is geared toward the achievement of objectives. The process is designed to identify events that could affect the enterprise and it manages those risks within its risk appetite. ERM is not an event or a circumstance, but a pervasive continuous series of actions that permeate the way management runs the business. It is not something added on to an enterprise's way of doing business—ERM is intertwined with the entity's operations and management. The basic framework is illustrated in Figure 6.6. The right face of the cube shows that risk management occurs across the enterprise. The top face illustrates the enterprise objectives that are served by ERM. The presenting face summarizes the steps in the process. Each cube face is discussed in turn below.

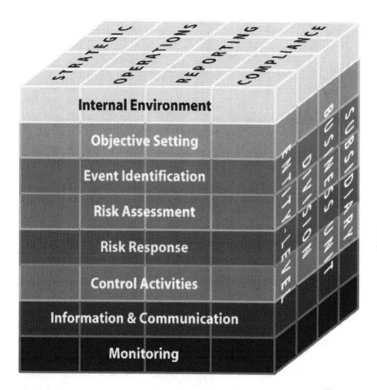

***Figure 6.6*** COSO ERM framework. (Copyright 2004 COSO. All rights reserved. Used by permission.)

## 6.8.1    *Across the enterprise*

ERM helps a firm's management select strategy consistent with the company's risk appetite. Risk appetite is the amount of risk a firm will accept in pursuit of value. Different strategies expose the entity to different risks. For example, pursuit of foreign markets is a high-risk position in which to put one's self. Conversely, failure to pursue foreign markets may severely limit a firm's profits and growth. A firm's risk appetite guides its resource allocation. Management allocates resources across business units in consideration of the firm's risk appetite and the individual business units' strategies for generating a desired return on invested resources (COSO, 2016). Management considers its risk appetite as it aligns its organization, people, and processes, and designs infrastructure necessary to effectively respond to and monitor risks.

Successful ERM requires an entity to consider its entire scope of activities. Every division, business unit, and subsidiary (see right face of Figure 6.6) must be engaged in risk management. That means there is a risk management hierarchy. ERM encompasses the entire scope of the firm's activities. This includes enterprise-level activities like strategic planning and resource allocation and business unit activities like marketing, production, new customer development, special projects, and new initiatives that might not yet have found a home in the firm's structure.

Most ERM frameworks, including COSO's, require a portfolio view of risk. This gives rise to the Rubik's Cube structure of the framework. Each business function in the entity (right face) has objectives (top face) and must follow the ERM process (presenting face) assessing the risk for each function or unit. It is management's responsibility to manage the entity's overall risk portfolio to ensure it is commensurate with its risk appetite. This requires them to consider interrelated risks from a portfolio perspective. Risks for an individual purchase decision, for example, may be within the unit's risk tolerances, but taken together with other purchases, they may exceed the risk appetite of the firm as a whole. In a portfolio view, management considers potential events to understand how they can affect the enterprise.

## 6.8.2   Achievement of objectives

Risk is defined by COSO as the possibility that events will occur and affect the achievement of strategy and business objectives. ERM is designed to achieve an entity's strategic, operational, reporting, and compliance objectives. These distinct categories of objectives overlap, that is, a particular objective may address different needs and could be the direct responsibility of several executives. Strategic objectives include the firm's high-level goals that are aligned with and support its mission. Operations objectives assure the effective and efficient use of the firm's resources. Objectives relating to reliability of reporting and compliance with laws and regulations are within the firm's control, so ERM should be reasonably assured of meeting those objectives. Strategic and operations objectives are influenced by external events that make their achievement more uncertain. The key idea, at this point in the discussion, is that ERM permeates the firm's vertical and horizontal structure and the objectives of each of those elements. This is what makes ERM enterprise wide.

## 6.8.3   Components of COSO's ERM framework

Figure 6.7 provides an effective summary of the nuts and bolts of the COSO ERM framework. There are eight interrelated ERM components derived from and integrated with the way management runs an enterprise. The ERM process begins by understanding the firm's internal environment,

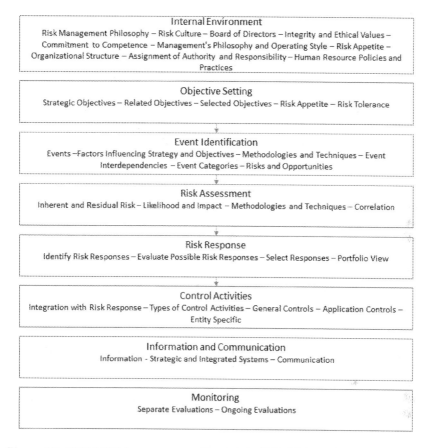

**Internal Environment**
Risk Management Philosophy – Risk Culture – Board of Directors – Integrity and Ethical Values – Commitment to Competence – Management's Philosophy and Operating Style – Risk Appetite – Organizational Structure – Assignment of Authority and Responsibility – Human Resource Policies and Practices

**Objective Setting**
Strategic Objectives – Related Objectives – Selected Objectives – Risk Appetite – Risk Tolerance

**Event Identification**
Events –Factors Influencing Strategy and Objectives – Methodologies and Techniques – Event Interdependencies – Event Categories – Risks and Opportunities

**Risk Assessment**
Inherent and Residual Risk – Likelihood and Impact – Methodologies and Techniques – Correlation

**Risk Response**
Identify Risk Responses – Evaluate Possible Risk Responses – Select Responses – Portfolio View

**Control Activities**
Integration with Risk Response – Types of Control Activities – General Controls – Application Controls – Entity Specific

**Information and Communication**
Information - Strategic and Integrated Systems – Communication

**Monitoring**
Separate Evaluations – Ongoing Evaluations

*Figure 6.7* COSO ERM components. (Copyright 2004 COSO. All rights reserved. Used by permission.)

which influences the risk consciousness of its people and provides discipline and structure for all other components of ERM. The internal environment comprises the firm's risk management philosophy, its risk appetite, and risk culture, among the other factors listed in the figure. This internal environment shapes and influences strategies and objectives, how business activities are structured, and how risks are identified, assessed, and managed.

Objectives must exist before they can be achieved. Every firm faces risks from a variety of external and internal sources. Which of these risks will be assessed and responded to depends critically on the firm's objectives. Strategic objectives provide a basis for establishing operations, reporting, and compliance objectives. When these objectives are aligned with the firm's risk appetite, they drive the risk tolerance levels for the company's activities.

Internal and external events that can affect achievement of the firm's objectives must be identified. Then management identifies the risks of loss and opportunities for gain among them. These and other events with potential negative or positive impacts on the firm's objectives will require management's assessment and response. It is important that management consider the full scope of the organization when identifying events that could influence achievement of organizational objectives. Likewise, management must recognize the uncertainties that can influence these events.

Firms undertake risk assessment to anticipate the extent to which potential events might impact the achievement of objectives. Both the likelihood and consequence of the risk needs to be assessed using either qualitative or quantitative methods. The positive and negative impacts of potential events need to be assessed across the enterprise. The likelihood and consequence of risks that emerge from the identified events are analyzed to form a basis for determining how they should be managed.

The firm chooses whether or not to respond to the risks that have been assessed. Management can accept, avoid, reduce, prevent, share, or live with the assessed risk, according to the firm's risk tolerance and risk appetite. Costs and benefits can be expected to weigh heavily in the firm's response. The risk that remains after a risk response is implemented, that is, the residual risk, should be assessed. This enables the enterprise's risk managers to bring the expected likelihood and consequence of a risk within the firm's risk tolerances.

Control activities are the policies and procedures enterprise risk managers put into place to ensure the risk responses are carried out. With ERM, control activities occur at all levels and in all functions of the organization. They can include changes in business processes, production process changes, compliance changes, and so on. A single control activity could help achieve firm objectives in several categories.

Information is needed at all levels of an organization to run a successful business. Likewise, information is needed to identify, assess, and respond to risks. Businesses use their internally generated data and information about external events to manage enterprise risks. Effective risk communication requires that all personnel receive a clear message from top management that ERM responsibilities must be taken seriously. Each person must understand their own role in ERM, as well as how their role affects or is affected by the work of others. Firms need an effective means of communicating information upstream and they must establish effective communication with external parties. All of this information must flow in a form and time frame that enables everyone to carry out their ERM responsibilities.

ERM decisions must be monitored to assure that the desired effects on objectives are being achieved. This is ordinarily done through ongoing monitoring activities or in separate evaluations. A firm's ERM framework changes over time. Risk responses that were once effective may become irrelevant. Control activities may become less effective, or no longer be performed. The firm's objectives may change. Management needs to determine whether existing ERM measures continue to be effective, in the face of such change, and to respond accordingly.

## *6.9  Three enterprise risk management concepts*

It is important to note once again the genesis of ERM in the for-profit business sector. The terminology was generated there to meet the needs of that sector. As is often the case, terms generated for a specific context can be appealing to those laboring in a different context. The terms are adopted, adapted, and the confusion begins. Efforts to adapt the ERM language to government and nonprofit sectors have been hampered by an inability to seamlessly translate some of the key concepts of ERM to these new contexts. This has led to no small amount of confusion about the meaning of these terms. The Internet is rife with explanations that point in many conflicting directions.

As with all other terminology turf battles, there is no illusion that they can be resolved here. It is, however, important to be clear about what the terms mean as they are used here. Three key terms have been selected for discussion, they are risk profile, risk appetite, and risk tolerance. Risk appetite and risk tolerance are frequently incorrectly interchanged. A solid understanding of the definition of these related yet different concepts has eluded the greater Internet community, despite the confidence of each individual source of information. Perhaps this discussion should begin with some caveat emptor. Here is my short take on these concepts. A risk profile is an objective representation of an organization's overall exposure to a group of risks at a given point in time. Risk appetite is an entity's policy for taking risk. Risk tolerance defines the upper and lower limits on risk that will initiate a risk response. Each of these concepts is discussed in the pages that follow.

### *6.9.1   Risk profile*

A risk profile is, at a minimum, a description of a set of risks of concern to an organization. This description can extend to a high-level assessment of the types of risks an organization faces. It is a representation of an organization's overall exposure to some specific risk or group of risks at a given point in time. The purpose of a risk profile is to provide an objective understanding of an organization's enterprise level risks.

A risk profile is quite different from a risk assessment; they are very different risk management tools. The risk profile is usually a high-level effort, conducted at the enterprise, business unit, product, or branch level. It may be closer to a risk prioritization process than to a risk assessment, which, by contrast, has a narrower focus and is more detailed and specific. The outputs are intended for different purposes. Risk profile results identify high level areas of risk that require management attention, which may include additional assessment of the risk. A risk assessment focuses on the consequence and probability of a risk and how effective risk controls can be against that risk. The familiar green, amber, red heat map or risk matrix is a common tool for conducting a risk profile.

The risk management team should be able to measure the gaps between the organization's risk profile and its risk appetite to understand the organization's risk landscape. An effective risk profile reflects the nature and scale of the entity's risk exposures across each relevant risk category.

## 6.9.2   Risk appetite

The risk appetite guides the enterprise in determining the types and amount of risk it is willing to accept in pursuit of its strategic and business line objectives. Every organization must take risks to achieve its objectives. The critical ERM question is how much risk do they need to take? Taking risks without intentionally managing them can lead to the organization's failure. The COSO ERM Framework defines risk appetite as "the amount of risk, on a broad level, an organization is willing to accept in pursuit of stakeholder value." ISO Guide 73:2009 defines it as "the amount and type of risk that an organization is willing to pursue or retain." Risk appetite, therefore defines an organization's desired pursuit of risk. This includes its willingness to accept losses and its desire for upside risk.

The Internet is teeming with definitions and explanations of risk appetite. Unfortunately, it is not teeming with consistency. Aven (2012) provides an academician's review of some thirteen different definitions. He argues that effective use in practice requires clear and understandable concepts, noting that risk management struggles with the nomenclature, with a number of diverging ideas and conceptions of risk and related concepts in use. Different environments and people support different interpretations and this affects the use of the term "risk appetite." He argues that risk appetite should be used to express the entity's willingness to take on risky activities in pursuit of value. It is a term used for describing a policy for risk taking.

Afforded the opportunity to observe organizations in various stages of transition to ERM, a striking constant has been the quickness with which employees latch on to the notion of a risk appetite. They want to know from their bosses, how much risk can we take? Their motivations may be more concern for personal culpability than for the strategic objectives of the organization, but their need is transparently clear. They need the top management of the organization to take charge and articulate the risk it is okay to take.

An organization's risk appetite should be prepared by its top management. It then needs to be carefully communicated throughout the organization. There does not appear to be any fixed or defined format for a risk appetite statement. Appetites will vary depending on the sector, culture, and objectives of the organization. A range of appetites may exist for different risks within a single organization and these appetites may change over time or with circumstances. Typically, a risk appetite statement is provided for enterprise-level risks. Operationalizing the risk appetite for enterprise-wide risks requires that the appetite statements become more specific as one drills down into the layers of the organization.

For example, an organization may express a low risk threshold for human life, health, and safety throughout the enterprise. That appetite statement will be applied quite differently aboard an oil drilling rig than it would be in an office environment, although both operations would be tasked with protecting human life, health, and safety.

Examples of qualitative risk appetite statements for single risks from a variety of organizations follow:

- A computer gaming organization has a higher risk appetite for virtual reality products and is willing to accept higher losses in the pursuit of higher returns.
- A franchising organization has a low risk appetite related to risky ventures and therefore is willing to invest in new business but with low appetite for potential losses.
- A health service organization has a low risk appetite related to patient safety but a higher appetite related to response to all patient needs.
- A manufacturer of engineered wood products has adopted a higher risk appetite relating to product defects in accepting the cost savings from lower-quality raw materials.
- A government agency has a low risk appetite for life safety but a higher appetite related to transportation cost savings and ecosystem restoration benefits created.

- A liberal arts teaching college has a low risk appetite for teaching reputation and a moderate risk appetite for research reputation.

Quantitative statements of risk appetite are also common.

The organization is, then, expected to evaluate alternative strategies to bring its risk profile in line with its risk appetite as part of its ERM strategy. Strategies are evaluated in order to understand the potential efficacy and implications of the chosen strategy for the organization's risk profile. The RIMS 2017 ERM Benchmark Survey reported:

- 37% of respondents had an enterprise level risk appetite
- 15% of respondents had a business unit or divisional level risk appetite
- 8% of respondents had a departmental level risk appetite
- 49% have developed no risk appetite

There would appear to be room for considerable improvement in the use of the risk appetite.

## 6.9.3   Risk tolerance

The organization will define acceptable variation in pursuit of its strategic and business line objectives. Acceptable variation in performance is closely linked to risk appetite and is sometimes called "risk tolerance." Risk tolerance describes the range of acceptable outcomes for achieving a strategic or business line objective within the risk appetite. It also provides an approach for measuring whether risks to the achievement of strategic and business line objectives are acceptable or unacceptable.

Risk appetite identifies the level of risk the organization will pursue to meet its objectives. Inevitably, organizations may wander outside their appetites, but how far? Risk tolerance statements identify the specific minimum and maximum levels beyond which the organization is unwilling to go. These define the upper and lower levels of risk the organization can absorb without significantly impacting the achievement of its strategic objectives. Exceeding these limits triggers a risk response. Deviations within the expressed boundaries would be bearable, exceeding them would not be.

The COSO ERM framework says risk tolerance "reflects the acceptable variation in outcomes related to specific performance measures linked to objectives the entity seeks to achieve." ISO Guide 73:2009 defines it as the "organization's or stakeholder's readiness to bear the risk after risk treatment in order to achieve its objectives." These may do more to contribute to the confusion over this term than to clarify it.

Risk tolerance appears to be a relatively simple concept. Depending on the organization, it presents a series of limits that may be absolute in the sense that the organization will not exceed them or they may be thresholds that alert the organization to a breach of tolerable risks (IRM, 2011).

Tolerance levels can be depicted graphically as shown in Figure 6.8. Call all the risks the organization might face the risk universe. Risk appetite defines the subset of risks with which the organization wants to actively engage. Risk tolerance defines those risks, which if push comes to shove, the organization could reluctantly live with. In general, an organization with any options at all, wants to operate within its appetite and it will not exceed its tolerance. Or, exceeding its tolerance triggers an immediate risk response to return the organization within its tolerance, if not its appetite.

Examples of risk tolerances to match the risk appetite statements above follow:

- A computer gaming organization seeks an expected return of 20% on virtual reality investments, but is not willing to take more than a 25% chance these investments will lead to a loss of more than 25% of the organization's existing capital.
- A franchising organization will not accept more than a 5% risk that a new line of franchises will reduce operating earnings by more than 5% over the next 5 years.
- A health service organization will treat all emergency room patients within 2 hours and all critically ill patients within 15 minutes.
- A manufacturer of engineered wood products has targeted production defects at one flaw per 1,000 board feet.
- A government agency has a zero lives lost tolerance for the operation of its projects. It seeks an increase of two new transportation cost savings and ecosystem restoration projects per year over the next 5 years.
- A liberal arts teaching college expects to stay the same or rise in quality of teaching surveys, while it will accept up to a 10% decrease in its research rankings.

Risk tolerances are often easier to quantify than risk appetites.

Deloitte Touche (2014) presents a convenient way to think about these three concepts. Figure 6.9 is adapted from their work. Imagine a risk profile

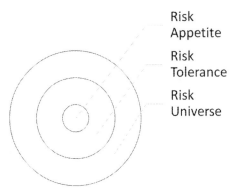

Risk
Appetite

Risk
Tolerance

Risk
Universe

***Figure 6.8*** Relationship of risk appetite and risk tolerance to an organization's risk universe.

that falls beneath the lower tolerance limit. Such an enterprise is not taking enough risk and corrective action must be taken. A risk profile that lands in the risk appetite area is in a desired position. A risk profile that is above the appetite but below the tolerance level has risks that have escalated beyond the desired range, corrective action can be expected. If the upper tolerance limit is exceeded by the risk profile, corrective action is required and risk must be reduced. Finally, if the risk profile exceeds the enterprise's risk capacity, the organization is no longer in a sustainable position.

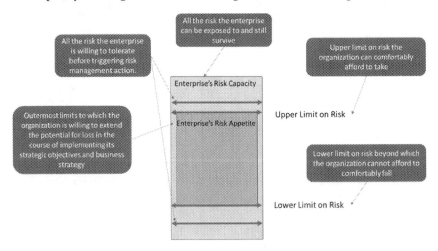

***Figure 6.9*** An enterprise's risk capacity, tolerance, and appetite. (Adapted from Deloitte Touche Tohmatsu Limited. 2014. Risk Appetite Frameworks, how to spot the genuine article. https://www.deloitte.com/content/dam/Deloitte/au/Documents/risk/deloitte-au-risk-appetite-frameworks-financial-services-0614.pdf (accessed April 13, 2018).)

## 6.10    Summary and look forward

ERM includes the methods and processes used by organizations to manage risks and seize opportunities related to the achievement of their objectives. Insurance and financial firms gave birth to ERM in the mid-twentieth century. ERM arises from a distinct business orientation that distinguishes it from other risk analysis and risk management models. Since its humble beginnings, ERM has spread rapidly to nonfinancial firms of all types and is now making inroads with many public institutions. One of its principle distinguishing characteristics is the buy-in of the Board of Directors and other top-level management of the firm who integrate risk management with the achievement of the organization's strategic objectives.

Two of the most popular risk management models are the COSO and ISO models. These models establish a standard and provide guidance for the conduct of ERM. Many alternative standards and models have been established for risk management.

Three important concepts of ERM were stressed: risk profile, risk appetite, and risk tolerance. A risk profile is an objective representation of an organization's overall exposure to a group of risks at a given point in time. Its risk appetite is likened to the organization's risk-taking policy and guidelines. Its risk tolerance defines the upper and lower limits on risk that will initiate a risk response. Although the language of ERM is quite distinctive, in principles and substance it is very compatible with the risk management model presented in Chapter 3. If you follow the process of that chapter, you will be practicing good risk management whether in an ERM, a public policy, or some other context.

Conscious attention is a scarce resource for decision makers so they tend to be selective about the information they use for decision making. If risk management is to succeed, we simply must find practical and effective ways to help decision makers become aware of and to account for uncertainty and the risks they give rise to in decision making. The next chapter, Decision Making Under Uncertainty, presents practical ways to do just that. It also includes an overview of several popular decision analysis techniques that are commonly applied in uncertain situations.

## References

Allianz Global Corporate and Specialty. 2018. *Allianz business barometer, top business risks for 2018*. London.

Aon plc. 2017. *Global risk management survey*. Aon Risk Solutions.

Aven, T. 2012. On the meaning and use of the risk appetite concept. *Risk Analysis* 33 (3), Doi: 10.1111/j.1539-6924.2012.01887.x

Barton, T.L. and J.B. MacArthur. 2015. A need for a challenge culture in enterprise risk management. *Risk Analysis* 8 (1); Fall.

Committee of Sponsoring Organizations (COSO). 2004. *Enterprise risk management: Integrated framework (2004)*. https://www.coso.org/Publications/ERM/ COSO_ERM_ExecutiveSummary.pdf (accessed April 13, 2018).

Committee of Sponsoring Organizations (COSO). 2016. *Enterprise risk management aligning risk with strategy and performance.*

Deloitte Development LLC. 2017. *Shift risk strategies, accelerate performance.* Risk and Financial Advisory, Fortune Knowledge Group.

Deloitte Touche Tohmatsu Limited. 2014. Risk Appetite Frameworks, how to spot the genuine article. https://www.deloitte.com/content/dam/Deloitte/ au/Documents/risk/deloitte-au-risk-appetite-frameworks-financial-services-0614.pdf (accessed April 13, 2018).

Deloitte Touche Tohmatsu Limited. 2018. *Global risk management survey*, 10th ed. Heightened uncertainty signals new challenges ahead. Deloitte University Press.

Fraser, J. and B.J. Simkins. 2010. Enterprise risk management an introduction and overview. In "Fraser, J. and B.J. Simkins (eds.), *Enterprise Risk Management Today's Leading Research and Best Practices for Tomorrow's Executives.* Hoboken: John Wiley and Sons.

Government Accountability Office. 2016. *Enterprise Risk Management Selected Agencies' Experiences Illustrate Good Practices in Managing Risk.* Report to the Committee on Oversight and Government Reform, House of Representatives. GAO-17-63.

Institute of Risk Management. 2011. *Risk Appetite and Risk Tolerance.* A consultation paper from the Institute of Risk Management.

International Organization for Standardization (ISO). 2018a. *ISO 31000:2018 Risk Management Guidelines.* Geneva: ISO.

International Organization for Standardization (ISO). 2018b. *ISO 73:2009 Risk Management — Vocabulary.* Geneva: ISO.

Kloman, H.F. 2010. A brief history of risk management. In J. Fraser and B.J. Simkins. (eds.), *Enterprise Risk Management Today's Leading Research and Best Practices for Tomorrow's Executives.* Hoboken, New Jersey: John Wiley & Sons.

Pergler, M. 2012. Enterprise Risk Management, What's different in the corporate world and why. *McKinsey Working Papers on Risk, Number 40.* https://www.mckinsey. com/business-functions/risk/our-insights/enterprise-risk-management-whats-different-in-the-corporate-world-and-why (accessed April 13, 2018).

Protiviti. 2006. Guide to Enterprise Risk Management, Frequently Asked Questions. http://www.ucop.edu/enterprise-risk-management/_files/ protiviti_faqguide.pdf (accessed April 13, 2018).

RIMS, Risk and Insurance Management Society. 2011. An Overview of Widely Used Risk Management Standards and Guidelines. https://www.rims. org/resources/ERM/Documents/RIMS%20Executive%20Report%20on%20 Widely%20Used%20Standards%20and%20Guidelines%20March%202010.pdf.

RIMS, the Risk Management Society. 2017. *2017 Enterprise Risk Management Benchmark Survey*, Executive Report. http://www.rims.org.

Surbhi, S. 2015. "Difference between public sector and private sector." *Key Differences.* May 20. https://keydifferences.com/difference-between-public-sector-and-private-sector.html (accessed December 29, 2017).

## chapter seven

# Decision making under uncertainty

## 7.1 Introduction

Judgments and decisions are often made intuitively rather than analytically. Decision makers draw upon personal memories, experiences, and associations that are supplemented by vast repositories of unconscious material that include cognitive biases and heuristics. They weave these materials together into explanatory stories that support their judgments and decisions.

Daniel Kahneman's (2011) work offers an explanation for how we formulate explanatory stories that we tell ourselves to give our world shape and meaning. We "humans," he argues, strongly prefer "fast" stories to "slow" logical processes and analytical judgments. He describes two discrete mental systems, System 1 and System 2, to explain this phenomenon. System 1 represents our fast, intuitive, and typically story-based decision-making and judgmental processes. It is also the dominant system that draws upon a blending of memories, associations, and quickly retrieved information to produce causal and associational thinking, which we use to create coherent explanatory stories upon which we base our judgments and decisions.

Unfortunately, System 1, although very fast and quite good at constructing compelling stories, is also prone to mistakes and systemic errors, especially so when we rely on biases and heuristics. System 2, by contrast, takes effort. It relies on laborious algorithms, probability, science, and evidence. System 2 can be used to monitor and "check" the accuracy of System 1 thinking, but it does not control System 1. The faster and intuitive System 1 typically dominates and it often prevails when the two Systems are at odds.

If decision making does not change with risk analysis then we have found its Achilles heel. It makes no sense to focus so much attention on the evidence and uncertainty in risk assessment if decision makers do not intentionally and carefully consider them during decision making. Risk analysis can be said to represent an effort to replace System 1 decision making with System 2 decision making.

In risk analysis, decision makers cannot count on the outcomes of their decisions. There is a range of outcomes and decision makers need to understand that. Risk is an important decision-making criterion. When risk is the only criterion, decisions are risk-based. When risk is an influential member of a set of decision criteria, decisions are risk-informed. In risk-based decision making, risk estimates and risk narratives form the basis for decisions. Unacceptable levels of risk trigger action. By contrast, risk-informed decision making trades off levels of risk with other criteria to arrive at a decision.

Risk analysis is a paradigm shifting decision-making framework. Analysts take great care to account for and document the potential effects of uncertainty on decision outcomes. Uncertainty is the engine of change here. In a decision-making context, it arises in one of two fundamental ways. First, the decision maker may not know the true values of one or more decision criteria because they are uncertain as a result of knowledge uncertainty, natural variability, or model uncertainty encountered while estimating those values. In these cases, decision makers must understand the resulting range of potential outcomes, what can cause those outcomes to occur, and their relative likelihoods. Second, the decision maker may understand the uncertainty inherent in the decision and just not know what to do in the face of that uncertainty.

Despite the best efforts of risk analysis, there is a mismatch between the clarity we hope the evidence can provide and the degree of certainty the evidence actually delivers. There is no shortage of methodologies for decision making under uncertainty. They range from elegant simplicity to impenetrable complexity. What the risk management community of practice needs is a practical approach, one that can be applied by decision makers with no special qualification beyond their interest in better decisions and better decision outcomes.

This chapter begins by considering the use of several decision-making strategies. The notion of risk analysis as evidence-based decision making is revisited in order to address one of the more perplexing paradoxes of decision making under uncertainty: how much evidence is enough to make a decision?; or, stated differently, how much uncertainty can a decision maker accept? Residual uncertainty is introduced as a formal topic to be considered by decision makers and to be communicated to decision makers. The chapter then turns its attention to offering a practical approach for decision makers who must decide under uncertainty. Finally, some more conventional approaches to decision making under uncertainty are presented before it concludes.

## 7.2 Decision-making strategies

Heuristics and bias research is usually said to have begun in the 1970s with the work of Tversky and Kahneman (1974). The research originally focused on the field of prediction under uncertainty and the estimation of probabilities and frequencies (Keren and Teigen, 2004). It did not take long for the research to be generalized to the whole area of judgment and decision making. Figure 7.1 presents the central elements of a decision process. There are the characteristics of the decision problem, which can be divided into the complexity of the decision task and the complexity of the decision context, the decision maker's goals and preferences, the decision strategy used, and the decision that is made.

The complexity of the decision task refers to the number of alternatives from which to choose and the number of attributes upon which to judge. The complexity of the decision context is affected by such things as the nature of the trade-offs entailed among the alternatives, the range of attribute metrics (alternatives with more similar metrics tend to be more difficult for decision makers to differentiate), and the quality of the alternatives and their similarities or differences.

The decision maker's goals can include such things as maximizing the accuracy of a decision, minimizing the cognitive effort required for the decision, minimizing the negative emotions experienced while deciding, and maximizing the ease of justifying a decision (Bettman, Luce, and Payne, 1998). The decision maker's preferences are important for determining attribute importance or weights, aspirational levels, that

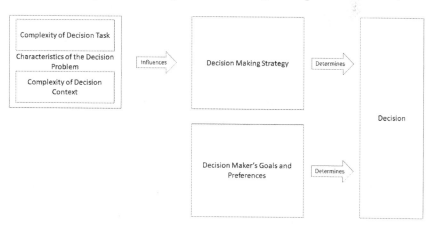

*Figure 7.1* Central elements of a decision-making process. (Adapted from Pfeiffer, J. 2012. *Interactive Decision Aids in e-Commerce.* Contributions to Management Science, DOI 10.1007/978-3-7908-2769-9 2, Berlin Heidelberg: Springer-Verlag.)

is, cutoff-values that identify thresholds or acceptable levels of an attribute, and value functions.

Decision making strategies vary by such characteristics as the amount of available information that is processed, whether trade-offs are considered explicitly or not, whether decision makers process information by alternative or attribute, the use of weights and/or aspiration levels, whether alternatives are screened in or out, the use of quantitative or qualitative data, and the like. All of these elements contribute to the decision that is made.

Risk analysis is evidence-based decision making under conditions of uncertainty. Classical economics relies on the notion of a rational decision maker, who possesses complete knowledge and has a stable set of preferences that are known well, along with sufficient computational skill to make decisions that achieve objectives, such as utility maximization, cost minimization, and profit maximization. Decision researchers increasingly see an alternative decision maker, one who constructs preferences and beliefs on the spot when needed rather than drawing on known, well-defined, and stable preferences (Payne and Bettman, 2004). These preferences are based on the use of a variety of decision heuristics. If we are going to influence decision making under uncertainty in a positive direction, it is incumbent upon us to understand something about the ways that decision makers process information.

Conscious attention is "the" scarce resource for decision makers (Simon, 1978). This means that decision makers will be selective about the information they use for decision making. Payne and Bettman (2004) point out that this highly selective decision processing does not necessarily mean poor decisions are being made. However, to the extent that decision makers attend to irrelevant information or neglect instrumental information, poor decisions can be made. Thus, it is crucial to help decision makers focus on instrumental information.

Simon (1955) introduced the idea that limited cognitive capacity requires the use of decision strategy heuristics that rely on selective and simple use of information to solve decision problems. The information processing approach to judgment and decision making assumes an individual possesses a set of such strategies, acquired through experience and perhaps formal training. Payne and Bettman (2004) conclude that heuristic methods for solving complex problems with limited information generally produce satisfactory outcomes. However, they can and do produce decision errors that tend to be systematic and predictable. So, let us examine some of the more common strategies people use to solve the classic multiattribute choice problem.

A multiattribute problem typically has a goal, such as to choose the best alternative and multiple (n > 2) alternative solutions from which to choose.

*Table 7.1* Comparison of characteristics of four information processing decision strategies

| Characteristic | Weighted additive strategy | Lexicographic heuristic | Satisficing heuristic | Elimination by aspects heuristic |
|---|---|---|---|---|
| Information used | All | Some | Some | Some |
| Explicit consideration of trade-offs | Yes | No | No | No |
| Basis for information processing | Alternative-based | Attribute-based | Alternative-based | Attribute-based |
| Attribute Weights | Explicit | Implicit | None | Implicit |
| Aspiration levels | No | No | Yes | Yes |
| Elimination of alternatives | No | Yes | No | Yes |

The decision is based on each alternative's contribution to a set of multiple (n > 2) attributes. Different people use different strategies. Some process information on multiple attributes for one alternative before moving to the next alternative, that is, they have an alternative focus. Others will examine the values of several alternatives for a single attribute before moving to another attribute, that is, they have an attribute focus.

Several such strategies are introduced in Table 7.1. Each is summarized in turn. The weighted additive strategy is often considered a normative rule for decision making. Each attribute measurement for an alternative is assigned a utility value, and those values are weighted by subjective weights assigned to each attribute and summed. The alternative with the maximum sum of utilities is the preferred option. This is a variation of the equal weight heuristic in which all attributes have the same weight; this is equivalent to a simple sum of the unweighted utilities. Multicriteria decision analysis methods would include the weighted additive method.

In the lexicographic heuristic, decision makers first consider the attribute with the highest importance. They select the alternative with the highest or an acceptable value for that attribute. If this produces more than one alternative, they iteratively compare the remaining alternatives for the next most important attribute. This process continues until there is only one alternative left. A related heuristic is the minimum difference lexicographic rule. The distinction here is that attribute values for two alternatives are considered to be equal if their difference is less than a value determined by decision makers. That value is based on a threshold above which a decision maker notices a difference between two attribute values. Thus, for example, cost estimates within $1,000 of one another might be considered equal costs. In another context, costs within $1,000,000 of each other might be considered equal.

With the satisficing heuristic, decision makers consider alternatives in the order in which they occur in the choice problem. The attributes of the first alternative are compared to the corresponding aspiration levels set by the decision makers for each attribute. Decision makers stop evaluating alternatives as soon as one of them meets all aspiration levels. If no alternative meets this criterion, the aspirational levels are reduced or new alternatives are formulated. With the satisficing-plus strategy, decision makers consider a subset of the attributes and the first alternative to meet their aspiration levels is chosen. The conjunctive strategy is based on the elimination of alternatives if they fail to meet the aspirational threshold of one or more attributes. Satisficing screens alternatives in, conjunction screens them out.

The elimination by aspects strategy begins with decision makers sorting the attributes from the most important (highest weight) to the least important. Starting with the most important attribute, alternatives are removed if the value of the alternative for that attribute does not meet the aspiration level. Those alternatives that pass the first round of evaluation are iteratively removed from consideration by considering the next most important attribute. The strategy continues until one alternative is left. If a unique choice is not reached, the aspirational levels can be adjusted.

It is clear that some of these heuristics conserve cognitive efforts. The lexicographic strategy is highly selective in the information it uses. Stopping after a satisfactory alternative is identified, in the satisficing heuristic, can save a lot of information processing. It is not uncommon to see decision makers use a combined strategy, beginning with an alternative eliminating strategy and then analyzing the remaining alternatives in more detail.

Payne and Bettman (2004) found that decision heuristics can be highly accurate with substantial reductions in cognitive effort but no one heuristic is accurate across all environments. Their research showed that decision makers increase their use of decision heuristics as the decision task becomes more complex. For example, when a decision offers many alternatives, decision makers tend to try to eliminate some of them as soon as possible. However, that strategy may shift to a more complex strategy as the number of alternatives decreases. Heuristics are especially useful when the decision maker is under time pressure. Most heuristics offer significant time savings over strategies like the weighted additive. In summary, they found that individuals use a variety of strategies to make multiattribute decisions, including heuristics that rely on highly selective information processing.

Payne and Bettman (2004) argue that our limited cognitive capacity requires us to use these mechanisms that involve the selective and simple use of information to solve decision problems. They further argue that we use these heuristics because they generally produce satisfactory outcomes. We may use them because there is no other option when our limited cognitive capacity or limited time for processing information act as constraints on our decision-making options. We may choose to use them because of the cost in time or effort of using our scarce resource of computational capacity or we may use them because they have worked in the past.

What we do know is that the rational decision maker of economic theory who follows the laws of logic, knows the calculus of probability, and is equipped with perfect information does not describe the way we make decisions. Most risk problems are intractable computationally, that is, we neither know the optimal solution nor a method for finding it. This opens the door to the use of fast and frugal heuristics. Fast means it can solve the problem quickly, within seconds even, and frugal means it requires little information. The early literature concluded that heuristics generally lead to second-best choices at best and irrational choices at worst. More recent literature suggests heuristics may do better than was once thought.

This chapter offers examples of rational decision making in Section 7.11. It should be used whenever possible. However, you are cautioned to bear in mind that real decision makers often rely on heuristics and biases that can influence judgments and decision making. This is especially true because decision making under uncertainty leads back to the roots of heuristic and bias research. Thus, it is important to get the most instrumental information in front of decision makers and to do a good job early in the risk management process of identifying decision criteria.

## 7.3   Evidence-based decision making

Most people agree that public policy should be based on the best available scientific and technical information. Many would agree that private sector decisions are, likewise, enhanced by facts and sound evidence. The central role of evidence in effective decision making is unassailable. Even so, it is not unusual for experts and decision makers to decide based on heuristics and bias or to have different interpretations of what the evidence means. The Council of State Governments (2013) offers six reasons why these differences in interpretation seem to emerge.

*Lack of Information*—Despite our access to vast and growing amounts of data and information, we rarely face policy problems with an obvious solution. Problems include not enough data; too much data to absorb; outdated data; restricted access to certain data; inconclusive data; data irrelevant to the decision at hand; existing studies have different objectives, assumptions, or methods of data collection and analysis; and insufficient analysis of the existing data.

*Lack of Agreement*—There can be fundamental disagreements about the information needed to inform a particular decision. Different parties may define the problem and objectives differently resulting in different conclusions about the information needed.

*Lack of Incentives*—The paradigm risk analysis would displace in public policy is an adversarial one that can pit science against politics and one interest group against another. Adversarial advocates cherry-pick their evidence in order to prevail in the process. There is little interest in resolving their differences in an evidence-based manner. Adversaries are adept at exploiting existing uncertainty and incomplete understanding is often touted as a reason for delaying decisions. The adversarial use of science can undermine trust in science, experts, and the decision-making process.

*Lack of Capacity*—Some stakeholders may lack access to data due to the lack of scientific and technical resources or because of data confidentiality. Stakeholders differ in their expertise and ability to understand the data. Different stakeholders can be expected to have different tolerances for risk and uncertainty.

*Lack of Communication*—A fundamental lack of communication and understanding among experts, decision makers, and advocates can give rise to disputes. Scientists may be interested in different issues than decision makers and stakeholders. Participants may have unrealistic expectations of the experts, science, and the ability to predict the future.

*Media Hyperbole or Oversimplification*—Conflict sells. Some media may overemphasize minor disagreements and make the issue look out of proportion. Writers may lack the technical background necessary to discern details or nuance when summarizing a story or gathering information on a debate.

In light of these reasons for regarding the evidence in different ways, let us consider the nature of evidence and what makes for good evidence. Evidence has been summarized here as anything that helps assessors discern the truth about a matter of concern to them. Evidence, then, is factual information that helps the risk manager or other decision maker reach a conclusion and form an opinion about something. Evidence-based decision making embodies the modern view of scientific policy advice in which science informs policy by producing objective, valid, and reliable knowledge (Funtowicz, 2006).

Figure 7.2 presents an evidence hierarchy. The predictive power of the decision increases as the supporting evidence moves up the hierarchy. Decision Innovations (https://www.decision-making-solutions.com) defines the evidence hierarchy categories as follows:

- Analogical evidence is a weak form of evidence that suggests something true about one thing is also true about another thing due to its similarity.

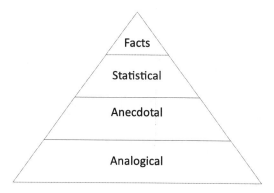

*Figure 7.2*  Evidence hierarchy.

- Anecdotal evidence arises from small sample sizes that are frequently not representative of typical experience. Anecdotal evidence indicates possibility without establishing likelihood.
- Statistical evidence provides evidence of causality, but it does not prove causality. Statistical inference helps establish causal relationships.
- Facts represent verifiable actual occurrences. They include empirical and historical evidence as well as scientific facts that can be confirmed with repeatable experiments.

The legal system, which has already done a great deal of careful thinking about evidence, provides a second way to consider evidence. In general, it identifies four types of evidence:

1. Real evidence, which includes tangible things
2. Demonstrative evidence, which may include a model of what likely happened at a given time and place
3. Documentary evidence, like reports, letters, and other documents
4. Testimonial evidence, which comprises witness testimony

The basic prerequisites for admissible evidence are that it be relevant, material, and competent. These are also reasonable requirements for risk analysis. Evidence is relevant if it has a tendency to make a fact more or less probable than it would be without the evidence (Federal Rules of Evidence, Rule 401 https://www.law.cornell.edu/rules/fre). Evidence is material if it is offered to prove a fact that is at issue in the case. Evidence is competent if it tends to prove the matter in dispute. These are qualities decisions makers would value as the judiciary would.

## EVIDENCE AND CONFIDENCE

When making decisions under uncertainty, decision makers should take care to understand and appreciate the strengths and weaknesses of the evidence upon which a decision will be based. Relevant material and competent evidence free the decision maker to rely more confidently on the facts than they can absent such evidence.

There are several other terms that can be profitably borrowed and adapted from the legal field. Evidence that tends to prove a factual matter by proving other events or circumstances from which the occurrence of the matter can be reasonably inferred is called circumstantial evidence. Evidence that is independent of and different from but that supplements and strengthens evidence already presented as proof of a factual matter is called corroboratory evidence. Hearsay evidence can be described as a statement offered as proof that what is stated as true is true. Hearsay is usually deemed inadmissible as evidence. There is a rule of evidence, the exclusionary rule, that excludes or suppresses evidence obtained improperly.

Although these notions were developed for a different field of inquiry, this is not a bad lexicon for risk assessors to borrow from. Examine each bit of information to assure its provenance and use only evidence that are relevant, material, and competent.

Now, let us turn our attention to the nature of this evidence and how it becomes useful for decision makers. Russell Ackoff (1989) is credited with being among the first to represent the knowledge hierarchy as a pyramid. Figure 7.3 presents a stylized data, information, knowledge,

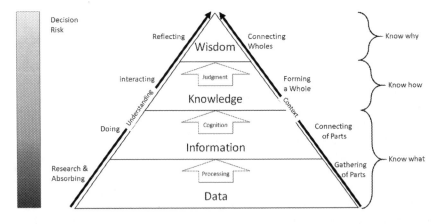

*Figure 7.3* DIKW pyramid mashup of two other pyramids.

wisdom (DIKW) pyramid that is a mashup of a U.S. Army Knowledge Managers pyramid (Wikipedia, 2018a) with a pyramid developed by Karim Vaes (2013).

Data are raw facts that have no meaning of themselves. Data simply exist in a usable or unusable form. Ackoff (1989) describes data as symbols that represent the properties of objects and events. Rowley (2007), who studied the DIKW definitions provided in textbooks, describes data "as being discrete, objective facts or observations, which are unorganized and unprocessed and therefore have no meaning or value because of lack of context and interpretation." Truth and objectivity are fundamental properties of data and facts, so incorrect facts or false data are precluded from this definition. A spreadsheet database full of peak daily streamflow measurements at a specific gage location is an example of data. Data are gathered through research or absorbed from the world around us.

Ackoff (1989) says information consists of processed data where the data have been processed specifically to increase its usefulness. Thus, information is data that has been given meaning by way of some relational connection. Rowley (2007) describes information as "organized or structured data, which has been processed in such a way that the information now has relevance for a specific purpose or context, and is therefore meaningful, valuable, useful and relevant." In contrast to Rowley's structural definition of information, Henry (1974) defined information as "data that changes us." Using the streamflow data to produce a flow-frequency curve is information. Information is gained by doing something with data.

Knowledge is the collection of relevant information with the intent to be useful (Wikipedia, 2018b). It can also be described as the synthesis of multiple sources of information over time. Thus, knowledge is a deterministic process. Someone must put forth effort to acquire knowledge and this knowledge has useful meaning to the seeker. Knowledge is sometimes described as information connected in relationships. Using the information from flow-frequency and depth-flow curves, analysts can develop knowledge about the depth and frequency of flooding in a town. Knowledge is gained by combining information in interactive ways.

Ackoff (1989) describes wisdom as the ability to increase effectiveness. Wisdom requires judgment and it adds value. Knowledge and understanding are commonly conflated in discussions of the DIKW pyramid. The values implied by knowledge are inherent to the analyst and are, therefore, unique and personal. Wisdom can ask questions to which there are no easily-achievable answers. Wisdom is the process by which we discern, or judge, between right and wrong, good and bad, ethical and unethical. Knowledge of a flood risk can lead to wisdom in managing that risk and preventing similar risks in the future through flood risk management measures and land use controls.

Understanding is a cognitive and analytical process that runs throughout the wisdom building process, it includes processing, cognition, and judgment. It facilitates movement from one tier to the next. Understanding is the process by which we recognize information in data, it is how we construct knowledge from information, and, perhaps most importantly, it is how we take existing knowledge and synthesize new wisdom from it. Understanding facilitates useful action.

Risk analysis would aspire to turn as much evidence into wisdom as possible. Decisions are not made based on data. The pursuit of data for the sake of its completeness is the equivalent of a false god for those who pursue evidence-based decision making. What risk managers need is wisdom. What risk assessors can best provide is the information, knowledge, and understanding necessary to give birth to that wisdom. When we speak of gaps or holes in our data, the real concern is how those holes affect the information that is available to us to construct the knowledge required to give birth to wise decisions.

> When making decisions under uncertainty, decision makers are well-advised to understand where the decision critical evidence rests in the DIKW pyramid. Proven knowledge is more valuable than raw data and speculation.

## 7.4   How much evidence is enough?

Gathering information in the face of uncertainty is a rational response by decision makers. Information gathering includes reading newspapers, books and journals, doing research, consulting experts, taking a class, conducting surveys, doing additional analysis of the available data, and the like. The common sense behind this approach is obvious. If we can reduce uncertainty about future outcomes we can make better choices (Clemen and Reilly, 2014).

Our minds are not comfortable with uncertainty. Most of us experience uncertainty as a threat that needs to be reduced, resolved, or overturned, the less uncertainty the better. Uncertainty implies doubt and danger. It is random and volatile. When information is missing, our brains say, "Uh-oh, what if this is important?" Risk assessors and analysts must be able to differentiate between questions worth exploring and questions best left unasked or at least unanswered. It is easy, even natural, to overestimate the value of missing data. Some individuals and organizations are obsessed with filling information gaps and that obsession can lead them astray, especially today, when so much information is so accessible.

Decision making under uncertainty is best served by a systematic and consistent approach to risk management. This begins by carefully establishing the decision context. That means identifying problems and opportunities, specifying objectives and constraints, formulating questions that risk assessment or other analyses need to answer, and identifying decision criteria. All of these tasks are best done at the outset and iteratively throughout a risk management process. A strong foundation in the decision process goes a long way in defining the questions that are necessary to answer. Limiting the questions a risk management activity pursues is the first and best way to limit the amount of data and information collected.

This brings us to the crux of one of the most important issues related to uncertainty. For the questions you need to answer, how much information is enough? Stated equivalently, how much uncertainty is too much? Or, when is the best time to make a decision?

Assessors may, at times, struggle with the appropriate level of detail in a risk assessment. Reducing uncertainty always has a cost. So, what is the appropriate level of detail? The answer is at once simple, elegant, and not terribly pragmatic; the level of detail shall be sufficient to make the decision at hand. Do not pay to gather evidence that is not needed to make a good decision. Built into this concept of an appropriate level of detail is an implicit notion that the risks associated with not reducing the uncertainty further have been considered.

Decision making needs to be grounded in reality. It cannot be based on default positions, consensus, what the boss believes, unsubstantiated opinions, whim, or fancy. "What is the evidence of that?" is an important question to ask repeatedly throughout the decision process. We live in a world of resource constraints and we cannot do everything. Thus, we must make choices about what evidence we will and will not pursue in a risk assessment.

Figure 7.4 demonstrates the basic trade-off between the costs of reducing uncertainty through evidence gathering and the amount of uncertainty that remains.* A good evidence gathering strategy is to gather only the evidence needed to make the risk management decision. The shape of the curve makes it clear that the only way to reduce evidence-gathering costs is to live with more uncertainty. The only way to reduce uncertainty is to devote more resources to evidence gathering. A good risk management process that establishes realistic expectations of the risk assessment and other analyses is the best way to address this trade-off.

Gathering data is wasted time, money, and effort if it does not add relevant evidence in the form of information, knowledge, and wisdom to

---

* The figure, as drawn, suggests zero uncertainty may be possible. This is not always the case.

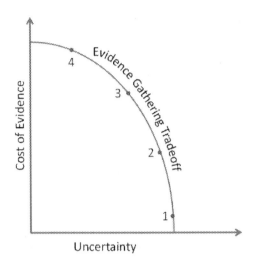

*Figure 7.4* Trade-off between evidence gathering cost and uncertainty remaining. (From Yoe, C. 2017. *Principles of risk analysis for water resources.* U.S. Army Corps of Engineers, Institute for Water Resources.)

our decisions. We call a piece of information relevant if it could impinge on the decision in some, even subtle, way. Relevant information may make one RMO look more appealing than another, or it might make a stakeholder happier. Relevant information can be categorized as instrumental or noninstrumental (Bastardi and Shafir, 1998). The ability to distinguish between the two is essential to both good risk assessment and good risk management. To be faithful to the language of Bastardi and Shafir's argument, "information" is used below, but "evidence" would work as well.

Instrumental information is a piece of information that can alter the decision that is made or the outcome of a decision. This would include decision criteria and other things one needs to know in order to make a decision. Noninstrumental information refers to information that would have no instrumental value if it were directly available. That is, these data may be, in some way, relevant and of interest but they would not affect the decision to be made or its outcome once it is made.

The contradictory conundrum is that noninstrumental information can come to acquire instrumental mystique once it has been sought. Analysts are rarely aware of pursuing noninstrumental information, instead, they may pursue this information because it appears or is believed to be relevant to the decision at hand. Then, having spent time, money, and effort pursuing the data, analysts or decision makers treat the information as instrumental and may even proceed to make their decision partly on the basis of this noninstrumental data. Bastardi and Shafir (1998) point out that whereas the information would have had no impact on the decision had it been directly available, the act of pursuing it can lead people to make choices they would not otherwise have made.

Thus, some individuals and some organizational cultures are prone to gather too much data, data that do not produce higher levels of knowledge on the pyramid or data that produce information that is not needed for decision making. In a world of scarce resources and limited budgets, it makes sense to only gather the information that is needed to make a decision and to accept the remaining uncertainty as relevant noninstrumental information.

A former student offered the following example. I do not know the height of my vehicle, it is uncertain. I do know I am about six feet tall and my vehicle is just below my shoulders. So when I approach a bridge that is 14 feet high, I do not have to do any more work to figure out the height of my vehicle, it is uncertain but reducing it further will not affect my decision. However, if I am driving a truck and I guess its height to be between 13 and 15 feet, it is going to be well worth my time to stop and measure as I approach that bridge.

Having more evidence may reduce your anxiety, but, unless it changes your decision, it is not worth the cost of obtaining it. Ask yourself, "Could this additional evidence affect the decision?" If the answer is no, forget it. If the answer is yes, then ask how likely it is to change the decision? If the possibility is remote, you may not need the evidence. Do not pursue evidence to perfect your decision; pursue it when it might affect your decisions.

## 7.4.1   There is a best time to decide

How much evidence do you need to make a decision? Let us reframe that question for the moment as "What is the best time to make a decision?" and consider it further. Some decisions, like whether to read a journal article or not, require minutes to make, others, like what is the proper scale of a risk management response to a major social problem, may take years to make.

Consider Figure 7.5 to help visualize the competing forces at work. Imagine a perfectly scalable relationship. As analysts spend time and money to increase their evidence base and knowledge, they are adding value to decision making as they increase their confidence. If analysts take

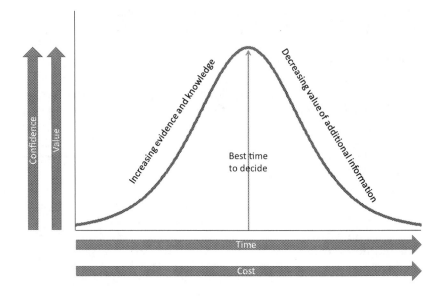

*Figure 7.5* Optimal time to make a decision. (Adapted from Decision Innovation (http://www.decision-making-solutions.com/decision-timing.html)

too much time and spend too much money, the value of the additional information decreases.

The point to take from this conceptual figure is that there is a best time to make a decision and that time comes before all the evidence has been collected and weighed. The image helps us visualize the competing forces at work when trying to find the best time to reach a decision. Too little time and the decision is made without knowledge that could have enabled a more informed and confident choice. Too much time and the benefits from the alternative solutions may be delayed, costs might rise, and in the case of some problems, losses or pain may continue to increase.

Risk managers may decide too soon by falling into one or more of the following traps (Decision Innovation, http://www.decision-making-solutions.com/decision-timing.html):

- Impulsive decision making or shooting from the hip
- Planning fallacy—underestimating how long it takes to get things done
- Primacy effect—weighing initial events, for example, decisions made in early iterations, more than later ones
- Risk neglect—the inclination to ignore risk when making uncertain decisions

- Herd instinct—the common bias of adopting the views of the majority
- Reliance on heuristics, rules-of-thumb, and other shortcuts

On the other hand, risk managers may decide too late by falling into these traps:

- Paralysis by analysis—seeking information that cannot affect the outcome
- Focusing on the analytical process rather than on its result
- Review anticipation—trying to preempt negative comments by trying to provide every bit of information conceivable
- Procrastination—waiting too long to begin actually deciding
- Risk register complacency—failing to actively manage high and medium risks to prevent their occurrence
- Maintaining the status quo—doing this analysis the way past analyses were done
- Job security—analysts continue analysis for as long as possible
- Lack of experience—results in mistakes and delays that delay the schedule and expand the budget
- Fear of litigation—drives the desire to gather additional information
- Normalcy bias—failing to respond effectively to an event, delay, or failure that has not happened before or that was not incorporated
- Fear—someone will criticize a mistake or missing data so information gathering is prolonged
- Vertical team failure—decisions previously made by the team are not subsequently honored, resulting in delay

Figure 7.5 shows the optimal point for making a decision occurs at the balance point between taking sufficient time to obtain the required knowledge to decide effectively and avoiding the loss in information value due to delaying the decision. As you might suspect, finding this optimum in practice is more art than science.

Difficult and highly complex decisions often lead to information gathering efforts that can have a serious negative impact on decision timing. The key is to gather enough information to get as close to the conceptual optimum decision-making data point as possible. This means reducing uncertainty strategically and gradually and deciding not when all uncertainty is reduced but when confidence and evidence enable a reasonable decision. Decision Innovation (http://www.decision-making-solutions.com/decision-timing.html) offers three specific strategies to help strike this balance. First, begin with lower cost exploratory efforts for decision options with high levels of knowledge uncertainty. Do not necessarily set out to eliminate uncertainty, begin by reducing it to the point where a decision can be made with a tolerable risk. Second, make the decision and proceed along the preferred decision path, but put checkpoints in place that would enable a new or revised decision based on knowledge gained through decision execution. Third, take actions to reduce the undesirable consequences of delaying a decision.

Too much emphasis on information gathering may interfere with effective decision making. Knowing enough to decide is critically important but knowing too much can clog up our cognitive processes. A complex set of regulations, such as some organizations rely upon, may cause decision makers to manage to the rules, if only for fear of falling afoul of them. Abundant policy and guidance documents can induce professionals to act defensively, focusing on the small print at the expense of the bigger picture. These defensive actions reduce risks to the decision makers but they are potential risks to decisions and the stakeholders they were intended to serve. Bloated budgets and swollen time frames can threaten the implementation and efficacy of risk management options.

We need information to both reduce the risk of decisions and to understand the risk in decisions but getting too much information can have real costs. In an active shooter situation, if we wait to gather more data then people may die; if you are buying a house and wait to gather more data about the neighborhood then the house could be sold before you act. Additional data do not increase information at the same rate, the marginal utility of another month, week, day of data decreases even as costs and time to gather that data rise. Most decisions can be and are made without all the information. Your best defense against premature or delayed decision making is a good strong risk management process.

## 7.5   Classifications of uncertainty

The uncertainty that remains after the best possible analysis has been done is called residual uncertainty (Courtney et al., 1997). Each risk management activity begins with significant amounts of uncertainty. A good risk management process will establish a comprehensive strategy to reduce uncertainty in a cost-effective and efficient manner. When the analysis ends and efforts to further reduce uncertainty have ceased, the uncertainty that remains is residual uncertainty. Three classifications of uncertainty relevant to decision makers are offered below.

According to Riesch (2013) there are several options for representing uncertainty. They are:

- Deny uncertainty or risk
- Concede there is some more or less undefined uncertainty
- List possible outcomes, qualitatively or quantitatively
- Provide likelihoods of the possible outcomes
- Provide statistical summaries and description of the uncertainty
- Provide a probability distribution

The representation people chose may depend on the point people want to make. In some instances, it may reflect philosophical stances or implicit assumptions made.

Decision makers must be aware of the level of residual risk in their decision problems in order to avoid adopting a dangerous binary view of uncertainty, that is, the world is predictable or it is not. A number of scholars have proposed categories or levels of uncertainty. Courtney et al. (1997) define four levels of residual uncertainty.

Level 1 is a clear enough future. While confident of the general shape of the future, we do not have precise values for some key variables. Decision makers have a single forecast of the future that is sufficiently narrow to point in a single strategic decision. The forecast is precise enough for decision making and the residual uncertainty is, for the most part, irrelevant.

Level 2 consists of a few discrete alternative futures. There are a variety of future outcomes, but we can list them and they are mutually exclusive and collectively exhaustive. Analysis cannot identify which outcome will occur, although it may help establish probabilities for the outcomes. The possible outcomes are discrete and clear but it is difficult or impossible to predict which one will occur. The decision strategy would change if the outcome became predictable.

Level 3 residual uncertainty comprises a range of futures that is defined by a limited number of key variables. The eventual outcome could lie anywhere along a continuum of possibilities. The range of potential outcomes is so numerous there are no natural discrete scenarios. Scenarios that can be constructed, like an optimistic or pessimistic case, are more representative of the many possible scenarios than they are unique scenarios of interest. The best decision strategy could change if the outcome became more predictable.

Level 4 is characterized by multiple interacting dimensions of uncertainty that make it virtually impossible to predict an outcome. The situation is so fluid and so unstable that it is impossible to even frame scenarios. Unlike level 3, the range of potential outcomes cannot be identified. In fact, it might not even be possible to identify, much less predict, all the relevant variables that will define the future. Level 4 is rare and these situations tend to migrate toward one of the other levels over time. Nevertheless, they do exist. The four levels are depicted visually in Figure 7.6.

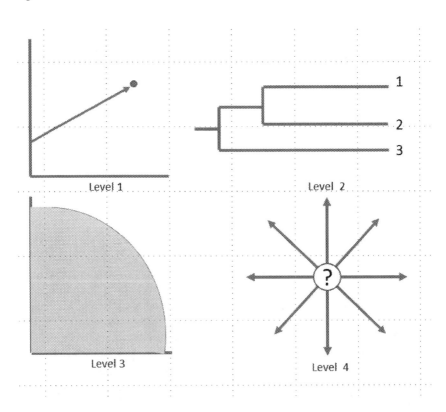

*Figure 7.6* Four levels of uncertainty defined by Courtney et al. (1997).

Courtney et al. (1997) have suggested that at least half of all decision problems fall into levels 2 or 3, while most of the rest are level 1 problems. They note that executives who think about uncertainty in a binary way tend to treat decision problems as if they fell into either levels 1 or 4. Perhaps most unsettling, those executives are most likely to apply the same set of analytic tools regardless of the level of residual uncertainty they face. Consequently, an important starting point for all decision makers is to understand the magnitude of the residual uncertainty in the outcomes of their decision problem.

Three types of decisions are identified by Courtney et al. (1997) as relevant for decision-making under the four conditions of uncertainty above. They are big bets, options, and no-regrets moves. Big bets are large commitments that will result in either large payoffs or large losses. Big bets are employed as shaping strategies (see text box). Options involve modest commitments that can be ramped up or scaled back as uncertainties are resolved. No-regrets moves pay off no matter what happens. Decision makers who are more sophisticated about decision making under uncertainty will be aware of the residual uncertainty and the types of decisions they face in their decision problem.

## SHAPING STRATEGIES

Courtney et al. (1997) identify three distinct strategic intents for decision makers under uncertainty. Shapers aim to drive the futures of their industries toward a new structure of their own devising. Adapters take the current industry structure and its future evolution as givens, and they react to the opportunities they are given. Those who reserve the right to play make incremental investments to preserve the option to decide and then wait until the environment becomes less uncertain to make a decision.

Walker et al. (2013) build on these ideas and define five levels of uncertainty bounded by complete certainty and total ignorance, as seen in Figure 7.7. The authors state there are many quantitative approaches for dealing with levels 1 to 3 uncertainty. Levels 4 and 5 comprise deep uncertainty (see text box) with level 4 being the "do not know" portion of the definition and level 5 uncertainties being the "cannot agree upon" portion of the deep uncertainty definition. There are fewer effective means for dealing with deep uncertainty.

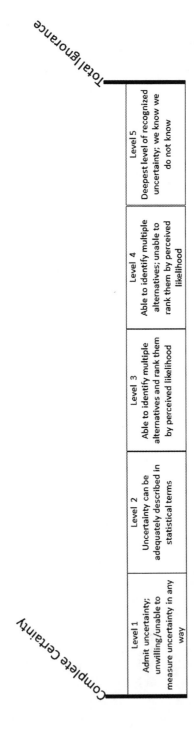

*Figure 7.7* Walker et al.'s (2013) five levels of uncertainty.

Lempert et al. (2003) define deep uncertainty as "the condition in which analysts do not know or the parties to a decision cannot agree upon (1) the appropriate models to describe interactions among a system's variables, (2) the probability distributions to represent uncertainty about key parameters in the models, and/or (3) how to value the desirability of alternative outcomes." The authors use the language "do not know" for individual decision making and "do not agree upon" for group decision making.

Riesch (2013) offers his own five-level classification of uncertainty. Level 1, is uncertainty about the outcome. This occurs when the model is known, the parameters are known, and the model predicts a specific outcome with a probability $p$. Level 2 is uncertainty about the parameters. We know the model but its parameters are not known. A quantity may be normally distributed but its mean and standard deviation may be unknown. Level 3 is uncertainty about the model. Models are usually simplifications about how the world works, and there are often several ways of modeling any given situation. Level 4 is uncertainty about known inadequacies and implicitly made assumptions. There are inevitable limitations to even the best models. Level 5 is uncertainty about unknown inadequacies. This is where we do know what we do not know.

## 7.6   Strategies for deciding in deep uncertainty

It is not likely that risk managers will master any of these classification systems but they may be of interest to those who want to think more carefully about uncertainty, especially for the purposes of helping decision makers laboring under uncertainty to choose a strategy for addressing it. Decision makers facing significant uncertainty often ask the wrong question, "what will happen?" instead of which actions available today are likely to serve best in the future? Several overlapping strategies for dealing with deep uncertainty (levels 4 and 5 from the above classification systems, which have no useful probabilities) are identified below (Reeves, 2016; Walker et al., 2013). These are:

- Classical—traditional approach of analysis, planning, and execution that basically ignores uncertainty and assumes one can rely on this information
- Resistance—plan for the worst-case scenario

- Resilience—choose a solution that results in quick system recovery no matter what happens in the future
  - Redundancy—buffers against unexpected events
  - Diversity—multiple ways of thinking and doing things as a hedge against change and to form the substrate for experimentation and learning
  - Modularity—firebreaks stop problems in one part of the entity from affecting the whole
  - Adaptation—learn and evolve by leveraging diversity in the face of change
  - Prudence—embrace unexpected upsides, while designing decisions to be robust to plausible unfavorable scenarios
- Adaptive robustness—prepare to change the policy in case conditions change
- Static robustness–choose a solution that performs reasonably well in practically all conceivable situations
- Adaptive management-use research, experiments, test plots, trial and error, and so on to reduce uncertainty to better inform managers before risk management options are irreversibly implemented
- Visionary—in a malleable environment, envision and realize new possibilities
  - Shaping—in both malleable and unpredictable environments, entities orchestrate the decision ecosystems using new business models
- Renewal—when viability is threatened, business models must be decisively transformed
- Precautionary principle—use discretionary decision making when the possibility of harm is not firmly established by the science

The classical response to uncertainty is nonviable. Resistance is usually costly and it may not perform well against black swans. Resilience accepts negative system performance in exchange for the ability to recover quickly. Static and adaptive robustness do not identify an optimal solution. Instead they provide a satisfactory level of performance across myriad potential futures. This stands in contrast to an optimal solution that achieves the best possible results but only across a narrow set of circumstances. Static robustness seeks to satisfice over a range of identifiable futures, while adaptive robustness adapts to changing conditions over time.

Adaptive management is a series of steps that promotes intentional learning about a problem and its potential solutions for the explicit purpose of reducing uncertainty to avoid irreversible errors or costly revisions to projects. In newly created, disrupted markets or other malleable environments organizations must be ready to seize opportunities. Shaping strategies are discussed in a preceding text box. When supply shocks, demand conditions, regulatory change, or competitive developments threaten the viability of organizations then new business models may be needed. The precautionary principle implies a social responsibility to protect the public from exposure to harm when scientific investigation has identified a plausible but largely uncertain risk.

The best risk managers will want to understand their residual uncertainty and the strategies available for responding to it. Such risk managers are likely to be rare for the foreseeable future so the responsibility for informing them may fall to the astute risk assessor.

## 7.7 Communicating uncertainty to decision makers

Preventing a false sense of certainty may be the single best reason for making decision makers aware of the uncertainty that attends their decision making. We need to banish that traditional approach of ignoring uncertainty to the dustbin of history. It is simply not sustainable. If we are to inform decision makers about uncertainty, it is wise to ask what decision makers want to know about uncertainty?

Relatively little research has been done on this topic, but Wardekker et al. (2008) provide a starting point. They report that policymakers participating in a survey have expressed the sentiment that assessment reports should not contain every nuance of uncertainty but should present only the most relevant uncertainty messages. Focus on instrumental uncertainties.

Survey takers said that uncertainty information may be used to:

- Assess the effectiveness and efficiency of policy measures more realistically
- Argue for one's own conclusions and against those in opposition
- Weigh information and the risks of using information that may turn out to be incorrect
- Determine the desirability of actions
- Estimate the plausibility of scenario's and trends
- Develop a vision on future government policies

Wardekker et al. (2008) point out that knowing about uncertainty has its drawbacks. It can make negotiations more difficult and it can weaken policy proposals. Decision makers can use it to argue in support of their own conclusions and against proposals that do not suit their interests or agenda. Too much uncertainty information could paralyze decision making through unnecessary discussion and delay of action. The general public may be confused by the complexity added by uncertainty information.

Decision makers identify three main areas where they would like more uncertainty information. These are:

- Topical issues that have received media attention
- Issues where uncertainty plays an important role but where there is little to no uncertainty communication
- Matters that are important for finding, selecting, and prioritizing policy responses

The policy relevance of uncertainty information was found to increase when:

- Being wrong in one direction carries more serious consequences than being wrong in the other
- Uncertain outcomes can have a large influence on policy advice
- Indicators are close to a policy goal or threshold
- Large effects or catastrophic events are possible
- There is societal controversy
- Value laden choices may conflict with the interests or views of stakeholders
- Public distrust in outcomes that show low risk can be expected

Uncertainties can be present throughout the risk management process beginning with the initial identification of a problem. It should come as no surprise that risk assessors and risk managers approach and regard uncertainty quite differently. Decision makers appear to be less interested in the extensive lists of uncertain values and the taxonomies of their source and type than in the direct implications of the uncertainty for decision making.

Textbooks and journal articles are filled with frameworks that tend to overengineer the decision-making process. Many existing frameworks for decision making under uncertainty are both comprehensive and complex. Their comprehensiveness tends to make them too complex and time-consuming to fit routine decision making. Experience teaches us that decision makers do not need more advanced techniques for making decisions under uncertainty, especially if we expect risk management to become increasingly more mainstream. Decision theory provides a useful and important set of tools that are quite appropriate for certain kinds of decisions. However, the vast majority of decisions being made in enterprise risk management organizations and in regulatory settings do not often fall into those categories of decisions. Most decision makers simply need some help wading through the flood of uncertainty that increasingly accompanies decisions. Consequently, what is needed is a good, common sense, practical approach to making decisions under uncertainty.

## 7.8   A practical approach

Uncertainty is an inevitable fact of life that can significantly limit the extent to which evidence can provide knowledge. Wardekker et al. (2008), adapting the work of Van der Sluijs et al. (2005), suggest a four-point scale of archetypes of attitudes toward uncertainty that are encountered in the decision-making world. These are:

- Avoid—Uncertainty is unwelcome and is to be avoided. Science is challenged to eliminate uncertainty by means of more and better independent research.
- Quantify—Uncertainty is unwelcome but unavoidable. Science is challenged to quantify uncertainty and to separate facts and values as effectively as possible.
- Deliberative—Uncertainty presents chances and opportunities. Science is challenged, by the existence of uncertainty, to contribute to a less technocratic, more democratic public debate.
- Science as player—The distinction between science and politics is artificial and untenable. Science is challenged to be an influential player in the public arena.

A survey by Wardekker et al. (2008) showed that a majority of policymakers held the "quantify" view with a sizable minority taking the "deliberative" view. The majority of scientists in the survey identified as deliberative with a sizable minority as quantify. Some policy makers and scientists identified with "science as a player," and a few scientists identified with "avoid." The remainder of this chapter adopts the quantify archetype.

The best leaders know how to make decisions in extremely uncertain circumstances and to keep moving forward (Johnson, 2015). Johnson offers a practical suggestion for decision making under uncertainty: get comfortable with the unknown. Humans want to reduce uncertainty and seeking more information sometimes feels like progress, when in fact, it can be a delaying tactic when the information we really need does not exist or is so difficult or costly to find that we cannot get it in time. He argues that decision making under uncertainty is sometimes best served by a balance of information and instinct.

Decision makers are not always motivated to reduce uncertainty. A common reaction to uncertainty is still to ignore it and act as if it does not exist. We may do that because we do not recognize it, we do not consider it relevant to our situation, or because we have learned to live with it. If our minds are made up, new information might conflict with our decision.

## COPING WITH UNCERTAINTY

Lipshitz and Strauss (1997) identify three broad strategies for coping with uncertainty: reducing it, acknowledging it, and suppressing it. Tactics for reducing uncertainty include: collecting additional information, deferring decisions, extrapolating from available information, assumption-based reasoning, mental simulation and scenario building, improving predictability through shorter time horizons, selling risks to other parties, selecting one of the possible interpretations of equivocal information, control the source of variation through standard operating procedures, and constraining the external environment by incorporating critical elements into the organization. Tactics for acknowledging uncertainty include taking it into account when choosing a course of action, preparing to manage potential risks, including uncertainty as a decision factor such as with the minimax or regret criteria, choosing options with clear outcome probabilities. Tactics for suppressing uncertainty include ignoring or distorting undesirable information and coping with uncertainty symbolically by going through the motions of reducing or acknowledging it.

**Source: Lipshitz and Strauss (1997)**

A less common approach to uncertainty is to embrace it and use it creatively and innovatively. Look for ways that uncertainty might be used to create a new future and to unlock untapped potential. The discomfort created by uncertainty might make us explore options we would not have considered in its absence.

The most obvious action to take when confronted with uncertainty is to reduce it by seeking new information and increasing our knowledge. But, will the additional information enable you to make a better decision? The answer is not always yes. Johnson notes that making a decision is one way to reduce uncertainty even if the decision is subsequently proven wrong. An incremental approach to decision making is, therefore, one way to reduce uncertainty while avoiding the risks of one big decision.

At the outset of this chapter, two fundamental decision-making issues were identified with uncertainty. They included not knowing the true values of the decision criteria and not knowing what decision to make in the face of uncertainty. To meet these challenges, decision makers must be clear about the decision that is before them, they need to understand the risks associated with the decision options and the uncertainties that give rise to those risks. Then they need to make a decision. A practical approach to meet these challenges is proposed below. The steps in this practical approach are:

- Understand the decision to be made
- Understand the residual risks and residual uncertainty
- Ask clarifying questions
- Make a decision or not

Each of these steps is described below.

## 7.8.1 Understand the decision to be made

Decisions are hard because of four broad sources of difficulty (Clemen and Reilly, 2014): complexity, multiple objectives, competing viewpoints, and uncertainty. Complexity is related to the number of issues that arise in a decision setting. Decision makers can be overwhelmed by complexity, making it difficult to give appropriate consideration to each component of the decision. When facing multiple objectives, progress toward one objective could impede progress toward other objectives. Such decision problems will always involve trade-offs. Decisions get difficult when different values and perspectives lead to different conclusions. This source of difficulty becomes especially pertinent when the number of decision makers grows beyond one. Of particular interest in this chapter is the inherent uncertainty in a decision situation. Decision making under uncertainty begins with the decision(s) to be made. If that decision is not understood there is little hope of a desirable outcome. This simple process begins by clarifying the decision that needs to be made.

Understand the risk complexity of the decision. Are the instrumental risks explicit or implicit? Is there a single risk or are there many? Some decisions involve a single risk decision. These can be as simple as: should we cross the street now or as complex as what is an acceptable daily intake for a new food additive. The decision maker focuses on a single primary risk decision in these instances.

By contrast, some decisions are more risk complex. These may require risk managers to make many incremental risk management decisions before arriving at the primary risk management decision. Imagine, for example, developing an anti-terrorism strategy for a city, or developing a comprehensive water resource management plan for a region. Such decisions require complex risk management options that entail many risk decisions and risk management features before a final go or no-go implementation decision.

Finally, there is a class of decisions that may not even be characterized as risk management decisions. Business decisions are an obvious example of this class. Opening a new store, introducing a new product line, or reorganizing a division may seem far from risk characterizations by decision makers. Even so, there are going to be risks associated with many of these decisions. Decision makers need to have a good understanding of the risk complexity of the decisions they are tasked with making.

Pay attention to complexity and carefully examine what the decision entails. As just noted, even when presented with a seemingly simple go/no-go decision, there can be many implicit decisions embedded in the decision before you. Good risk management chooses the best risk management option from amongst an array of different options, most of which will consist of multiple measures. Each of these measures may bring its own issues, its own objectives, and its own stakeholders with varying perspectives. When you make a seemingly simple go/no-go decision, you are also making a decision about each of those issues, objectives, and perspectives. Some of them may be significant. Some of them may entail risks of their own. Consequently, it is imperative that a decision maker understands the full implications of the decision before them. You may be very comfortable with the presenting decision but have grave misgivings about deploying a specific feature of that decision. Explore the embedded decisions before deciding.

No consideration of a decision problem can be complete until the decision maker(s) understands the potential outcomes of their decision. Any half decent decision process will identify the expected outcomes of a decision, but that is just the starting point. Decision makers must understand the full range of potential outcomes from each decision alternative. If we pass this regulation, build this public works project, institute this new product line, what will happen? What else could happen? What do we want/expect the outcome to be and what else could it be as a result of making this decision? These questions need to be asked of each and every decision alternative the decision maker faces. Once the potential outcomes are understood, it is time to understand the residual risk and uncertainty.

A good risk management process will go a long way toward providing this information for you. A thoroughly established decision-context will provide a list of problems to solve and opportunities to attain; it will identify the risks relevant to the decision. There will be a set of objectives and constraints that define what a successful resolution of the problems and attainment of the opportunities will look like. These objectives and constraints define successful outcomes for decision making. An ever-present generic decision question is which of the risk management or decision options will best achieve the objectives and avoid the constraints. If a good risk management process has been followed, this information will be more readily available. Otherwise, it will have to be generated before a decision is made.

## 7.8.2 Understand the residual risks and residual uncertainty

Residual risk is the risk that remains after risk management options are implemented and functioning. Inherent risk minus risk reduced equals residual risk. Residual risk probably ought to be a decision criterion in every risk-informed decision, whenever it is available. Residual uncertainty is the uncertainty that remains when all the data collection and analysis are completed for a decision problem. Part of the consideration of residual uncertainty ought to be to understand how it might affect the residual risk that accompanies each decision option. There may or may not be additional options for reducing the residual uncertainty. With respect to the decision to be made, residual uncertainty may be irrelevant, relevant and noninstrumental, or relevant and instrumental. Instrumental uncertainties are those that could have an effect on the decision choice or on decision outcomes. In addition to residual risk, new risks may arise as a direct or indirect result of a decision for convenience we will consider them residual to the decision. Broadly construed, new risks also include transferred and transformed risks.

Uncertainty can exist in any part of the knowledge pyramid. There can be gaps in our data, our information, our knowledge, or our wisdom. Uncertainty about the value of a decision criterion tends to reside in the gaps in our data and information, uncertainty about what to do resides in our knowledge and wisdom. There is an evidence gathering process in every risk management activity. Its purpose is to identify the relevant knowns and unknowns about a decision problem. Risk assessors and risk managers then develop a strategy for reducing or at least characterizing the unknowns that are instrumental to the decision(s) to be made.

It is the risk assessor's responsibility to communicate the significance and source(s) of the residual instrumental uncertainty. It is the risk manager's responsibility to decide how to weigh that in the decision process. Risk assessors begin by identifying the relevant uncertainty in their input variables and they proceed by efforts to reduce that uncertainty and/or by characterizing the effects of the instrumental uncertainty on assessment outputs.

Let us illustrate with a very simple example that considers two different scenarios. Acme Cleaners is considering producing and selling a new line of vacuum cleaners and they would like to know how profitable this product would be. The presenting choice is whether to produce 500,000 vacuum cleaners or not. On the left of Figure 7.8 is a scenario where the quantity sold and the average cost per vacuum cleaner are uncertain. The uncertain average cost is depicted by the uniform distribution at the top of the center column. The uncertainty about the quantity is represented by the pert distribution in the middle of the center column. These are the

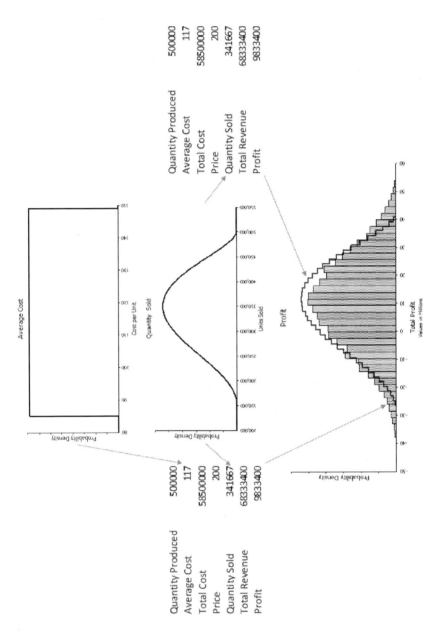

*Figure 7.8* A simple example with two uncertain input scenarios and two different output scenarios.

instrumental uncertainties. On the right is an alternative scenario where all inputs are known except the quantity sold.

The decision criterion is profit, which is shown in the bottom figure with two distributions, the instrumental risk is of a negative profit. Knowing the variation in outputs is important. Knowing why the outputs vary is also important. Communicating the uncertain inputs provides the decision maker with potential options. Imagine that a decision has to be made in the scenario on the left, with two uncertain inputs. The decision maker might have the option of negotiating a contract to solidify the costs of production, reducing cost uncertainty. This would reduce the profit uncertainty from the larger background distribution to the narrower foreground distribution. To reduce the uncertainty further, the decision maker could commission more detailed market research that might produce a more precise description of the uncertain quantity sold, than the pert distribution does. Knowing which inputs are uncertain can make a difference to decision makers. In other decision problems, knowledge of the uncertain inputs may be irrelevant to the decision.

Addressing the uncertainty in the decision criterion, profit, is solely the responsibility of the risk manager. The decision maker must know the range in potential outputs. In the scenario with two uncertain variables, a minimum profit of $-$40 million and a maximum of \$54 million with a mean return of \$9.8 million are all possibilities. A sensitivity analysis (not shown) indicates that the uncertain quantity sold contributes more to the variation in output than the uncertain cost.

It is useful to understand the likelihood of the various outputs and outcomes, especially those that could affect the decision choice. Clearly, decision makers will not produce the vacuum cleaners if the probability of a negative return is unacceptable. In the example, the probability of a negative outcome for the scenario with two uncertain inputs is 27.5% and it is 24.5% for the scenario with one uncertain input. Risk managers must now decide if this is an acceptable, tolerable, or unacceptable risk. Such thresholds may not always be so obvious for other decision criteria.

What new risks might be introduced by the decision choice? Language can be subtle, so let us point out that the range in model outputs is not necessarily the same as the range in outcomes. Outcomes can go beyond model outputs and decision criteria. What happens to Acme Cleaners if losses of \$40 million are suffered? Will the company remain viable? What happens to Acme Cleaners if they make \$54 million on the new product? Will it expand? What is the expected outcome? What will the company look like? What impact will this have on the company's strategic objectives? So, it helps if decision makers understand how decision criteria estimates and risk assessment outputs relate to outcomes of interest.

It is one thing to ask what the profit might be, it is an entirely different thing to ask what the outcome of different realizations of profit will be. Profit was the decision criterion in the example, but it is important to go beyond the outputs to think about the outcomes of interest. Considering the outcomes of a decision made under uncertainty amounts to conducting a simple risk assessment of the final decision choices. Consider new risks that might arise as a result of the decision choice. If we say yes to the production of 500,000 vacuum cleaners, what can go wrong? What are the consequences? How can it happen? How likely is it that they will occur? Are there potential outcomes we cannot live with? How likely are they to occur? These are all relevant considerations.

Residual uncertainty may be described narratively, qualitatively, or quantitatively. When the decision maker is presented with a range of outputs or decision criteria to consider, the decision implications of the entire range of values should be considered. For example, if the minimum value of −$40 million obtains what might the outcomes be? What decision would be made if the decision maker knew the minimum would obtain? If a five-number summary is used to display the uncertain results, the decision maker would repeat this process for the first quartile (−$1 million), median ($10 million), third quartile ($21 million), and maximum ($54 million) values as well.

Can the decision maker live with all the outcomes? Must some of them be avoided? Are there any feasible options for reducing the risk of their occurrence? Have they been included as part of the risk management options being considered? With Courtney et al.'s (1997) level 2 uncertainty, you have discrete outputs or alternative futures. Some of these will be more attractive than others. With level 3 uncertainty, there is more of a continuum of outputs as seen in the example above. At what point does the continuum become unacceptable? These are the sorts of understandings to seek about the residual uncertainty and the outcomes they can produce. It will often be the risk assessor's responsibility to facilitate this kind of analysis.

It is important for a decision maker to understand what further options there may be for reducing the residual uncertainty? How might the decision data be improved? How much can the accuracy of the decision data be improved? Will ranges be narrower? Will confidence be higher? What will it cost to reduce uncertainty further? How long will it take?

## 7.8.3  Ask clarifying questions

Unlike risk assessors, many risk managers are likely to be uncomfortable with uncertainty. As a result, it is important for decision makers to "wrap their heads" around the uncertainty and become comfortable with its implications for decision making. Uncertainty about decision criteria is more than a five-number summary, it includes the reasons for that spread in the data.

Once the decision maker has a sound understanding of the decision to be made and its residual risk and uncertainty, it is time to focus on reducing or at least understanding decision outcome uncertainty, a phenomenon quite different from the output uncertainty considered until now in this process. At its most fundamental level, decision outcome uncertainty appears when we do not know what the best decision is.

In situations where people may be reluctant to be transparent Brooks and John (2018) suggest that you ask yes or no questions to avoid evasive answers, then ask detailed follow-up questions to elicit more information. Ask the most sensitive question first so following questions feel less intrusive making people more forthcoming. Frame tough questions with pessimistic assumptions to reduce the likelihood that information is withheld. This risk "is likely to get worse before it gets better" will elicit more honesty than "you've got this risk under control, don't you?"

This is the time to clarify the range of outcomes that could result from the decision choices. If the decision outcomes differ from the decision criteria this needs to be carefully noted. Recall the example above where outcomes of interest to the Acme Co. could be distinguished from profit on the vacuum cleaner sales. The immediate goal is to make the potential results of the decision less confusing and more clearly comprehensible. Clarify the decision choices and their expected outcomes, then clarify the range of those expected outcomes and their probabilities. Clarify the causes of different outcomes, clarify the tipping factors and what causes an outcome to go from good to bad or from desirable to undesirable. Clarify thresholds and values that matter to you. What causes profits to be negative? What causes them to exceed $50 million? What makes costs jump over $70 million? What causes the revenue to exceed $70 million? What conditions have to be present? What is the likelihood that will happen? This is the time for decision makers to probe.

Following is a sequence of questions that could be used to start the process of clarifying uncertainty for decision making.

1. What is the decision that needs to be made?
2. What do we know with certainty?
3. What do we still need to know?
4. Do we have enough information to make this decision now?

5. What is the range of possible outcomes for this decision?
6. What combination of uncertain factors will result in a desirable outcome for this decision?
7. What combination of factors will result in an undesirable outcome for this decision?
8. How likely is a desirable outcome?
9. How likely is an undesirable outcome?
10. What are the risks associated with making this decision?
    a.  What can go wrong?
    b.  What are the consequences?
    c.  How can it happen?
    d.  How likely are those consequences?
11. What am I afraid of in making this decision?
12. What is the worst case, how likely is it?
13. Can I cope with the results of my decision?
14. Why am I making this particular decision?
15. Can I logically and honestly defend my decision?
16. Can I live with the risks that may be created, transferred, or transformed as a result of my decision?
17. What am I not asking you that I should?
18. Am I ready to decide?

### 7.8.4   Make a decision or not

This is a subjective step in the process. There is no foolproof way to make decisions, there is no recipe. When you are ready to make a decision, do so. If you are not, it may be time to escalate the decision to a higher authority. Document the decision rationale no matter how convinced you are that you will never forget it.

## 7.9   Practical changes

Introducing effective risk management to an organization is likely to present a monumental challenge. This section offers four early steps to take to implement the practical approach to risk-informed decision making described above. The steps are:

- To change the decision meeting
- Question the numbers
- Power down decision making
- Socialize errors that result from a good risk management decision-making process

## 7.9.1   Change the decision meeting

The best way for an organization to begin to change decision making is by changing the decision meeting. When a decision needs to be made, decision makers should come to the meeting prepared to make a decision. That means doing whatever preparatory work that needs to be done. To apply the simple process described above, decision makers should make sure they understand the risks that can affect the decision or the outcomes of the decision. Decision makers should ask their staff: If I make this decision, then:

- What can go wrong?
- What are the consequences?
- How can it happen?
- How likely are they?

Once the risks associated with a decision choice are understood, the decision maker must understand the uncertainty that can affect the decision or the outcomes of the decision. Decision makers can do that by asking:

- What is uncertain?
- Why is it uncertain?
- How uncertain is it?
- Why is the uncertainty important?

Forearmed with this information, the decision maker is better prepared to make a risk-informed decision.

## 7.9.2   Question the numbers

Risk analysis addresses the uncertainty inherent in decision making. That uncertainty needs to be adequately expressed to decision makers. It can range from a very simple and straightforward admission that we do not know the precise values of decision criteria to the presentation of probability distributions for decision criteria and everything imaginable between these two extremes. When a value is uncertain, it is important to characterize that uncertainty.

If risk managers are not presented with realistic summaries of uncertain decision criteria, it is incumbent upon them to question the numbers. Faced with making decisions under conditions of uncertainty, risk managers can do much worse than to make "there is no such thing as the number" their mantra. Point estimates of risky outcomes provide an illusion of precision that is not present. Point estimates of decision criteria derived from uncertain estimates of quantities can be misleading.

Many decision-making processes run on a single number. Analysts are trained to calculate it, decision makers adamantly insist upon it, the web master asks for it, financial systems require it to balance the books, and reporters want to know it. In a great many of these circumstances, "the number" is understood to be a "best estimate" or even a "best guess." To make decisions under uncertainty, decision makers must be well-informed about the uncertainty, the estimate, or the guess. Decision makers must take responsibility for becoming well-informed about the instrumental uncertainty.

One of the best ways to do this is to question the numbers with which they are provided for decision making. If given the number of individuals affected by a risk to health and safety, ask to see the distribution or a five-number summary. If one is not available, ask for realistic minimum and maximum values. If they have not been estimated, ask what circumstances could cause the minimum and maximum numbers to occur and how likely those circumstances are. If staff cannot answer those questions, then pose a scenario that could cause a lower and a higher value. Do what you must to find out what the true range of the risk estimates and other decision criteria could be.

Budgets are notorious for running on precise numbers. Estimating revenues or operating costs for the coming year is anything but a certain process. Give your staff permission to say they do not know for sure when uncertainty is present. Get comfortable with ranges and be very slow to accept a point estimate for any decision criterion without exploring its potential range of values.

### 7.9.3 Power down decision making

Highly effective organizations have leaders at every level, not just at the top. A third step to take to enhance an organization's ability to make decisions under uncertainty is to push down decision-making authority or to "power down." With risk-based and risk-informed decision making, outcomes may well matter more than chain of command or compliance with every bit of organizational guidance. Every risk an organization faces has or should have an owner who is responsible for actively managing that risk. A concerted effort to let the people closest to the outcome make the decision will be rewarded by better outcomes. These are the people who will be best informed about the risks, they will be closest to new information that can reduce uncertainty, and they are most readily available to manage these risks.

Organizations in a competitive environment may only have to reduce uncertainty a little faster than their opponent to gain a competitive advantage. The edge often goes to those who can learn quickly. Power down decision making and give less guidance. Pushing decision making down the organization, closer to the data, enables you to integrate more data into decision-making processes more quickly. The people closest to the job know it best. Do not slow the process down with excessive guidance and policy.

### 7.9.4 Socialize errors from good risk management

Managing risks means some things are not going to turn out as hoped. Bad outcomes should not be punished when they result from good risk management process. Berman (2015) suggests that organizations socialize the inevitable errors that will occur in risk management decision making. A culture of risk-informed decision making must be socialized. This includes both learning and teaching behaviors, beliefs and actions. If an organization follows good risk management practice, some undesirable outcomes will inevitably occur. Owners of these risks can learn from those experiences and the organization benefits from those lessons.

## 7.10 Risk metrics

Decision making under conditions of uncertainty may include yes or no decisions on a single action, rating a series of alternatives, ranking the alternatives, or choosing the best option from among a set of alternatives. It is the risk assessor's job to address the uncertain assessment inputs, to characterize uncertain outputs, and to convey the significance of the uncertainty in their assessments to risk managers. It is the risk manager's job to address the uncertainty in the assessment outputs and decision criteria and to take these explicitly into account in decision making. To do this, risk managers need to request and use risk information to aid in their decisions made under uncertainty. This means developing risk-related decision metrics. To the extent that risk managers become explicit about the risk metrics of interest to them, the decision-making process will be improved.

Typical risk metrics vary with the nature of the risks being considered in the decision context. They may include such things as mortality, morbidity, and life-safety risk, including such things as the number of lives at risk and social vulnerability. Relative risk, increases or decreases in risk, and odds ratios may also be used. Examples of other values at risk might include profits, net economic benefits, financial risks, engineering risk and reliability, and the like. The risks considered and their measurements should include the full range of existing risk, risk reductions, residual risk, risk transformations, risk transfers, and new risks as appropriate to the decision.

Risk-informed decision making is a new enough concept that the most useful risk metrics may have not even been identified as yet. Certainly, we have a good handle on the most obvious risk measures, and many of them have been in use for a long time. The emphasis on risk analysis, however, is young, and clever assessors will hopefully continue to develop new metrics to aid in decision making. One such metric is obtained from the partitioned multiobjective risk method (PMRM) developed by Haimes (1998). The PMRM was developed to respond to the common inadequacy of an expected value as a measure of risk. It develops conditional expected-value functions that represent the risk given that an event of a certain magnitude, frequency, or circumstance has occurred. The method can, for example, be used to isolate one or more damage ranges by specifying a partitioning probability. It then generates a conditional expectation of the consequences, given that the consequences fall within the identified range. An example follows.

Flooding is a serious risk to life and property in many parts of the world. Floods cause property damage and reductions in these property damages are a common measurement of the benefits to flood risk management measures. These damages are often estimated using the hydroeconomic model shown in Figure 7.9, which is used to estimate the expected annual damages (EAD) associated with flood regimes and flood risk management options.

Beginning in the upper-right quadrant, property damage is shown to increase as flood depths increase. Moving to the left, we see that increasingly large flows of water (measured in cubic feet per second) are needed to increase flood depths. Moving down a quadrant, the annual exceedance frequencies of these quantities of water are shown. The lower-right quadrant links the three relationships. Choosing any damage amount $a from the horizontal axis of the upper-right quadrant shows that damage is caused by b feet of water (upper left), which occurs with a flow of c cubic feet per second of water flow (lower left). That flow occurs with an annual exceedance frequency of d%, and so we have $a occurring with an exceedance frequency of d%. Such derived damage-frequency pairs ($a, d%) trace out the existing-condition damage-frequency curve. When the area under this curve is integrated, it yields an estimate of the expected annual damages (EADs).

The EADs for the example in Figure 7.9 are $12,411,000. The most common interpretation of this value is if the development in the flood plain and its hydraulics and hydrology remained unchanged for a long time (say 10,000 years) and we added the flood damages in constant dollars for each of these 10,000 years (most of these years would be zeros) and then divide the sum by 10,000, we would have an average annual damage of $12,411,000. This is a common flood-risk metric.

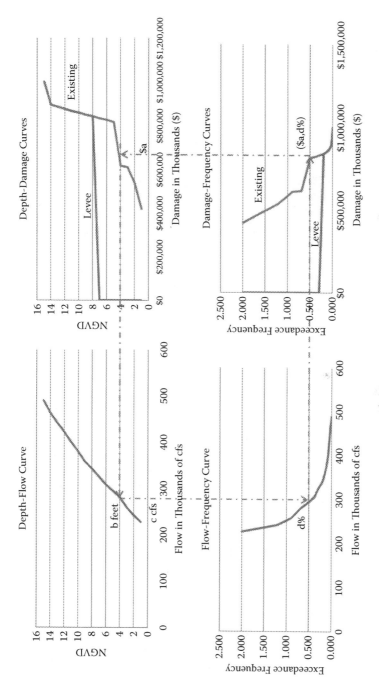

*Figure 7.9* Hydroeconomic model for estimating expected annual flood damages.

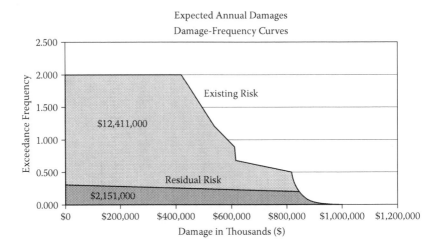

*Figure 7.10* Damage-frequency curves for existing and improved condition scenarios.

If this risk is judged to be unacceptable and it is to be reduced through a risk management option, the model in Figure 7.9 can be used to estimate the effectiveness of the risk management option (RMO). Most RMOs will alter one or more of the first three relationships in the model. A levee is shown in the upper-right quadrant of Figure 7.9, and its effect on the estimate of expected annual damages is shown in the lower-right quadrant, which is reproduced in Figure 7.10. Damages from floods up to seven feet in depth are reduced to zero by the levee. For the simplicity of the example, we ignore the risk of levee failure.

A levee is one option for managing the flood risk. Using the improved-scenario curve (levee) in place of the existing scenario, a residual risk damage-frequency curve is traced out for the levee, as shown in Figure 7.10. The area beneath this curve yields EAD of $2,151,000. This is a measure of residual damages. A measure of risk reduction is the difference between the EAD estimate for existing risk ($12,411,000) and residual risk ($2,151,000), in this case $10,260,000. This is the standard way of estimating the risk of property damage from flooding and of informing risk managers and the public about this risk.

EAD is now much lower, but what happens to the community when a flood large enough to overtop the levee occurs? Hurricanes Katrina and Rita, as well as flooding in the Midwest early in this century, have demonstrated the devastation that can result when levees fail or are overtopped. Risk partitioning is a useful tool for better informing risk managers and the public about extreme risks, and it is an example of a more creative risk metric to better inform decision makers.

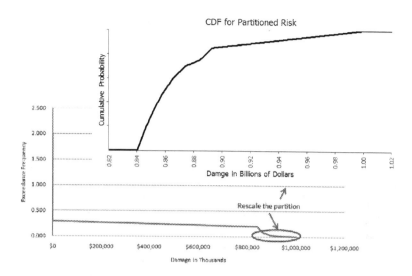

**Figure 7.11** A risk partition for the hydroeconomic estimation of flood risks.

Figure 7.11 illustrates the notion. Let us consider that a flood with an annual exceedance frequency of 0.002 or less occurs and overtops the levee. Now what is the expected value of damages? This is quite a different metric from the usual EAD. Haimes (2004) provides a rigorous treatment of this partitioned risk concept. In essence, it entails rescaling the probability (vertical axis) partitioned segment of the curve (circled) over the 0 to 1 scale and calculating the expected value of that new distribution. Recall that residual damages are $2,151,000. However, given that an event of equal or greater severity than the 0.002 exceedance frequency flood occurs, then the expected damages are $872,659,000. This provides an entirely different perspective on the residual risk. The likelihood of a flood overtopping the levee is low, but the consequences are devastating. This is not obvious from the more traditional measure of residual damages.

Different RMOs can yield different partitioned risks. For example, a channel or nonstructural flood risk management option might yield a lower traditional estimate of EAD reduced but also a much-reduced partitioned risk. Such risk metrics can provide valuable new insights for evaluating a flood RMO. The risk assessment community of practice needs to continue to develop and use clever and revealing risk metrics like this in all aspects of risk-informed decision making.

## 7.11 Decision analysis

There is no magic bullet coming. You will not learn a foolproof way of making a decision under uncertainty here because none exists. For all the helpful mathematics and science, decision making is still fundamentally an exercise in judgment. People weigh and choose. The methods they use for doing so may be formal or informal. Decision analysis, however, provides us with systematic approaches to decision making that reduces the likelihood of an uninformed decision.

Borrowing a definition from the *Business Dictionary* (www. businessdictionary.com) decision analysis is a: "Management technique in which statistical tools such as decision tree analysis, multivariate analysis, and probabilistic forecasting are applied to the mathematical models of real-world problems. The objective of a decision analysis is to discover the most advantageous alternative under the circumstances." Decision analysis can be used to develop an optimal strategy when decision makers have multiple decision alternatives and an uncertain future. Decision analysis is used to make better decisions, where better decisions are those that use a logical and coherent process that matches the decision maker's needs (Clemen and Reilly, 2014). Better decisions cannot guarantee good outcomes. Good decisions sometimes result in bad outcomes.

This section introduces the use of influence diagrams and decision trees in decision making. The treatment here is abbreviated because these topics are well-covered in the literature. The section begins with an example followed by considering some methods for making decisions under uncertainty without probability information. It then considers methods that can be used when probability information is available. The section concludes with a discussion of the value of information.

## 7.11.1 The example

Let us use a hypothetical example to develop the concepts and terminology of decision analysis. Silver Train Corporation (STC) purchased land that will be the site of a new luxury condominium complex in Sweet Virginia. STC commissioned preliminary architectural drawings for three different projects: one with 30, one with 60, and one with 90 condominiums. The financial success of the project depends upon the size of the condominium complex and the uncertain market demand for the condominiums. The STC decision problem is to select the size of the new complex that will lead to the largest profit given the uncertainty concerning the demand for the condominiums.

This decision problem is characterized by decision alternatives, states of nature, and resulting payoffs. The decision alternatives are the different possible strategies the decision maker can employ; in this case, the alternatives are building 30, 60, or 90 condos. The states of nature refer to future events which may occur that are not under the control of the decision maker. In this case, the states of nature are weak, moderate, or strong success, which depend on the demand for condos at the Sweet Virginia site.

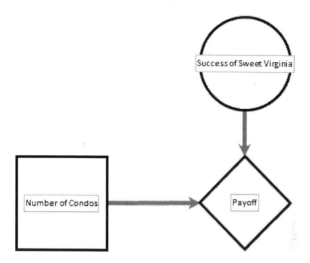

**Figure 7.12** Simple influence diagram for STC development of the Sweet Virginia project.

Figure 7.12 begins to explore this problem with an influence diagram. An influence diagram is a graphical device showing the relationships among the decisions, the chance events, and the consequences. Influence diagrams use several conventions:

- Squares or rectangles depict decision nodes
- Circles or ovals depict chance nodes
- Diamonds depict consequence nodes
- Lines or arcs connecting the nodes show the direction of influence.

The "Success of Sweet Virginia" node identifies the three states of nature and their respective probabilities. The "Number of Condos" node identified three decision alternatives and the "Payoff" node contains the payoff values.

The next tool is a payoff table derived from the influence diagram inputs. The consequence resulting from a specific combination of a decision alternative and a state of nature is a payoff. So, a 30-condo project with strong success returns $1,000, moderate success returns $500, and weak success breaks even at $0, as seen in Table 7.2. Other combinations of decision alternatives and states of nature have different payoffs. A table that shows the payoffs for all combinations of decision alternatives and states of nature is a payoff table. Payoffs can be expressed in terms of any appropriate measure; in this example, payoffs are the accumulated present value of all profits in thousands of dollars.

*Table 7.2* Sweet Virginia condo project decision analysis matrix

| Decision alternatives | States of the world ($ thousands) | | |
|---|---|---|---|
| Condominiums | Strong success | Moderate success | Weak success |
| 90 | $3,000 | $200 | ($2,000) |
| 60 | $2,000 | $400 | ($200) |
| 30 | $1,000 | $500 | $0 |
| | P(Strong) = 0.5 | P(Moderate) = 0.3 | P(Weak) = 0.2 |

## 7.11.2   Decision making without probability

We begin by considering decision making without probabilities. Five commonly used criteria for decision making when probability information regarding the likelihood of the states of nature is unavailable are:

- Maximax or optimistic approach
- Maximin or conservative approach
- Laplace criterion or equally likely approach
- Minimax or regret approach
- Hurwicz criterion

Maximax would be used by an optimistic decision maker. The decision with the largest possible payoff is chosen. In this instance, 90 condominiums provides the maximum payoff at $3,000. If the objective had been to minimize costs instead of maximizing profit and the payoff table showed the costs of the project instead of profits, the decision with the lowest cost would be chosen under this optimistic criterion.

The maximin approach would be used by a conservative decision maker. For each decision, the minimum payoff is listed and then the decision that yields the maximum of these minimum payoffs is selected. Hence, the minimum possible payoff is maximized. The 30-condominium project meets this criterion with a payoff of $0. If the objective and payoff were expressed in terms of costs, the maximum cost would be determined for each decision and then the decision that yields the minimum of these maximum costs is selected. Hence, the maximum possible cost is minimized.

The Laplace criterion considers all the payoffs for each alternative equally likely. In other words, each state of nature is assumed to have a 1/n chance of occurring, where n is the number of states of nature considered. In this event, each state of nature has a 1/3 chance of occurring. The criterion proceeds by finding the average payoff for each alternative and the alternative with the highest average is selected. Thus,

Table 7.3 Sweet Virginia condo project regret matrix

| Decision alternatives | States of the world ($ millions) | | | |
|---|---|---|---|---|
| Condominiums | Strong success | Moderate success | Weak success | Maximum regret |
| 90 | $0 | $300 | $2,000 | $2,000 |
| 60 | $1,000 | $100 | $200 | $1,000 |
| 30 | $2,000 | $0 | $0 | $2,000 |

the 90-condo alternative has a Laplace value of $400, the 60-condo value is $733, and the 30-condo value is $500. The 60-condo decision is best under this criterion.

The regret criterion requires us to construct a regret table or an opportunity loss table as shown in Table 7.3. This is done by calculating the difference between each payoff and the largest payoff for that state of nature for each state of nature. Strong success has a maximum payoff of $3,000. If the 90-condos option is chosen and strong success is realized, the regret for having chosen 90 condos is $3,000 – $3,000 = $0. However, if 60 condos had been chosen, the regret would be $3,000 – $2,000 = $1,000, and so it goes for all the table entries. Then, using this regret table, the maximum regret for each possible decision is listed. The option chosen is the one that minimizes the maximum regret; in this case, that is the 60-condo project with a maximum regret of $1,000.

An alternative approach is to use the Hurwicz criterion, sometimes called the criterion of realism or the weighted average. This criterion was developed as a compromise between the optimistic and pessimistic criteria. It requires the decision maker to select a coefficient of realism a, with $0 \leq a \leq 1$, such that a perfectly optimistic decision maker would set a = 1 and a perfectly pessimistic decision maker would set a = 0. The value for a represents the decision maker's coefficient of optimism and 1 – a represents their coefficient of pessimism. These two coefficients become the weights in the following equation:

Hurwicz value = a (Optimistic value) + (1 − a)(Pessimistic value).

Now, compute the weighted averages for each alternative and select the alternative with the highest value. Assume, for the sake of the example, the decision maker is rather optimistic and chooses a = 0.8, these values are:

90 condos: 0.8($3,000) + 0.2(−$2,000) = $2,000
60 condos: 0.8($2,000) + 0.2(−$200) = $1,560
30 condos: 0.8($1,000) + 0.2(0) = $800.

The best choice is 90 condos. A more pessimistic decision maker might well end up with a different ranking of the decision choices. The coefficient of optimism should not be confused with a probability value. Notice these criteria can and do provide different answers. There are no magic bullets.

### 7.11.3  Decision making with probability

Now we turn to decision making with probabilities and begin with the expected value approach. If probabilistic information regarding the states of nature is available, we may use the expected value (EV) approach (see Table 7.4). The expected return for each decision is calculated by summing the products of the payoff under each state of nature and the probability of that state of nature occurring. The decision with the best expected return is chosen.

The expected value of a decision alternative is the sum of weighted payoffs for the decision alternative. The expected value (EV) of decision alternative $d_i$ is defined as:

$$EV(d_i) = \sum_{j=1}^{N} P(s_j)(v_{ij}) \tag{7.1}$$

where: $N$ = the number of states of nature

$P(s_j)$ = the probability of state of nature $s_j$

$v_{ij}$ = the payoff corresponding to decision alternative $d_i$ and state of nature $s_j$

For this example, the expected values are shown in Table 7.4. Figure 7.13 presents the problem as a decision tree.

*Table 7.4* Expected values of STC's sweet Virginia development scales

| Decision alternatives | States of the world ($ thousands) | | | |
| --- | --- | --- | --- | --- |
| Condominiums | Strong success | Moderate success | Weak success | Expected values |
| 90 | $3,000 | $200 | ($2,000) | $1,160.0 |
| 60 | $2,000 | $400 | ($200) | $1,080.0 |
| 30 | $1,000 | $500 | $0 | $650.0 |
| | P(Strong) = 0.5 | P(Moderate) = 0.3 | P(Weak) = 0.2 | |

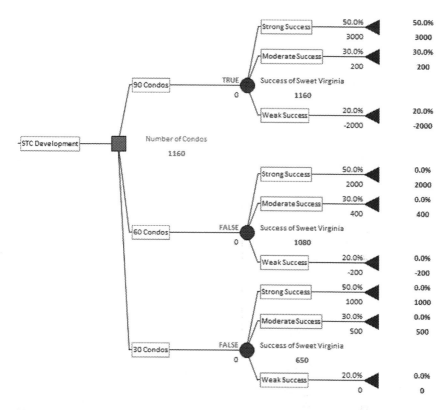

**Figure 7.13** Decision tree model of STC decision problem using expected values.

The tree shows the expected value of each chance event and the maximization objective identifies the 90-condominium project as the best option based on expected value, with a payoff of $1,160.

### 7.11.4   Risk profile and sensitivity

Risk analysis helps the decision maker recognize the difference between the expected value of a decision alternative, and the payoff that might actually occur. A risk profile* for the example is shown in Figure 7.14. It presents deviations from the expected value and shows the possible payoffs for the decision alternatives along with their associated probabilities. Notice the expected value of $1,160 is not one of the potential outcomes.

---

* As used here, "risk profile" is a Palisade PrecisionTree software feature that visually summarizes the potential consequences of an event tree. It should not be confused with previous definitions of that term. Risk language is messy.

Probabilities for Event Tree STC Development

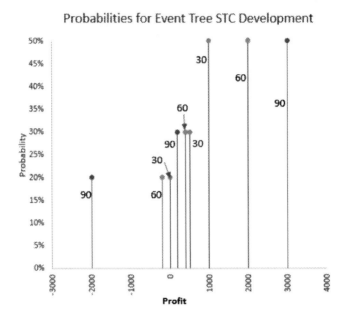

*Figure 7.14* Risk profile for STC development of Sweet Virginia.

A sensitivity analysis can be used to determine how changes to the tree inputs, that is, probabilities for the states of nature and values of the payoffs, affect the recommended decision alternative. Table 7.5 provides a sensitivity analysis for consequences. To read the table, look at step 3 of 90 Strong. If the input, that is, profit, rises from $3,000 to $3,750, this is a 25% increase. This results in a new output, that is, best expected value. It increases from $1,160 to $1,535, a 32.33% increase. If profit fell to $2,250, the best expected value would fall to $1,080, a 6.9% decrease. The 90-condo decision is reasonably robust across changes in profit. Notice that changes in the last five clusters of profit inputs do not affect the expected value because none of these changes is large enough to swing the best choice from the 90-condo option.

## 7.11.5   Value of additional information

Imagine that STC had the ability to consult a seer who could eliminate the uncertainty about which state of nature would be realized. What would that perfect information be worth to STC, that is, what is the expected value of perfect information? Frequently, additional information is available that can improve the probability estimates for the states of nature (or the size of the consequences if they are uncertain). The expected value of perfect information (EVPI) is the increase in the expected outcome, in this case,

**Table 7.5** Sensitivity of expected value to changes in consequences

Spider graph data

Decision tree "STC development" (expected value of entire model)

| Input name | Step | Input variation | | | Output variation | | |
| | | Value | Change | Change (%) | Value | Change | Change (%) |
|---|---|---|---|---|---|---|---|
| 90 Strong | 1 | 2250 | −750 | −25.00% | 1080 | −80 | −6.90 |
| | 2 | 3000 | 0 | 0.00% | 1160 | 0 | 0.00 |
| | 3 | 3750 | 750 | 25.00% | 1535 | 375 | 32.33 |
| 90 Weak | 1 | −2500 | −500 | −25.00% | 1080 | −80 | −6.90 |
| | 2 | −2000 | 0 | 0.00% | 1160 | 0 | 0.00 |
| | 3 | −1500 | 500 | 25.00% | 1260 | 100 | 8.62 |
| 60 Strong | 1 | 1500 | −500 | −25.00% | 1160 | 0 | 0.00 |
| | 2 | 2000 | 0 | 0.00% | 1160 | 0 | 0.00 |
| | 3 | 2500 | 500 | 25.00% | 1330 | 170 | 14.66 |
| 90 Moderate | 1 | 150 | −50 | −25.00% | 1145 | −15 | −1.29 |
| | 2 | 200 | 0 | 0.00% | 1160 | 0 | 0.00 |
| | 3 | 250 | 50 | 25.00% | 1175 | 15 | 1.29 |
| 60 Moderate | 1 | 300 | −100 | −25.00% | 1160 | 0 | 0.00 |
| | 2 | 400 | 0 | 0.00% | 1160 | 0 | 0.00 |
| | 3 | 500 | 100 | 25.00% | 1160 | 0 | 0.00 |
| 60 Weak | 1 | −250 | −50 | −25.00% | 1160 | 0 | 0.00 |
| | 2 | −200 | 0 | 0.00% | 1160 | 0 | 0.00 |
| | 3 | −150 | 50 | 25.00% | 1160 | 0 | 0.00 |
| 30 Strong | 1 | 750 | −250 | −25.00% | 1160 | 0 | 0.00 |
| | 2 | 1000 | 0 | 0.00% | 1160 | 0 | 0.00 |
| | 3 | 1250 | 250 | 25.00% | 1160 | 0 | 0.00 |
| 30 Moderate | 1 | 375 | −125 | −25.00% | 1160 | 0 | 0.00 |
| | 2 | 500 | 0 | 0.00% | 1160 | 0 | 0.00 |
| | 3 | 625 | 125 | 25.00% | 1160 | 0 | 0.00 |
| 30 Weak | 1 | −50 | −50 | − | 1160 | 0 | 0.00 |
| | 2 | 0 | 0 | − | 1160 | 0 | 0.00 |
| | 3 | 50 | 50 | − | 1160 | 0 | 0.00 |

profit, that would result if one knew with certainty which state of nature would occur. The EVPI provides an upper bound on the expected value of any additional sample or survey information undertaken to reduce the uncertainty about which state of nature is more likely.

Here is how it works. For each state of nature, select the highest payout and weight it by its probability, call this the value with perfect information

(EVwPI). It is $1,650 and is seen below. The expected value without perfect information (EVwoPI) is the decision alternative with the highest expected value, the 90-condo choice at $1,160. These calculations look like this for our example:

> Expected value with perfect information (EVwPI): 0.5($3,000) + 0.3($500) + 0.2($0) = $1,650
> Expected value of optimal decision without perfect information (EVwoPI): 0.5($3,000) + 0.3($400) + 0.2(−$2,000) = $1,160
> Expected value of perfect information (EVPI): $1,650 − $1,160 = $490.

It would be foolish to spend more than $490 (a year) for perfect information.

These are simple examples of some common applications of decision theory. Note, as mentioned earlier, the theory is far more sophisticated than has been demonstrated in this brief overview. Those interested in learning more should consider Clemen and Reilly (2014) *Making Hard Decisions with Decision Tools* for an introduction and Kochenderfer et al. (2015) *Decision Making Under Uncertainty Theory and Application* for a more complete treatment of the topic.

## 7.12  Summary

If risk assessment and its intentional focus on uncertainty do not improve decision making then the risk analysis sciences will have failed in a fundamental way. Risk analysis is decision making under uncertainty.

There are a great many sophisticated methods for decision making under uncertainty but many of them are simply not practical for most organizations that struggle with fundamental issues like how much analysis is needed to make a decision and how to get decision makers to consider uncertainty. To address these fundamental needs, this chapter has argued there is a best time to make a decision and a practical approach to making decision under uncertainty is needed. Four tasks are identified as a foundation for a practical approach. These are understanding the decision to be made, understanding the residual risks and residual uncertainty, asking clarifying questions, then making a decision or not. Four tactics to help initiate this process are: change the decision meeting, question the numbers, power down decision making, and socialize errors that result from a good risk management process.

## References

Ackoff, R.L. 1989. From data to wisdom. *Journal of Applied Systems Analysis* 15: 3–9.
Bastardi, A. and E. Shafir. 1998. On the pursuit and misuse of useless information. *Journal of Personality and Social Psychology* 75 (I): 19–32.

Berman, J. 2015. 3 Ways to take action in the face of uncertainty. *Harvard Business Review*. December 8, 2015. https://hbr.org/2015/12/3-ways-to-take-action-in-the-face-of-uncertainty.

Bettman, J.R., Luce, M.F. and Payne, J.W. 1998. Constructive consumer choice processes. *Journal of Consumer Research* 25, 187–217. http://dx.doi.org/10.1086/209535

Brooks, A.W. and L.K. John. 2018. The surprising power of questions, it goes far beyond exchanging information. *Harvard Business Review*. May–June 2018. https://hbr.org/2015/03/avoiding-decision-paralysis-in-the-face-of-uncertainty.

Clemen, R.T. and T. Reilly. 2014. *Making hard decisions with decision tools*. 3rd ed. Mason, OH: South-Western, Cengage Learning.

Council of State Governments, Sound Science Advisory Board. 2013. A State Official's Guide to Science-Based Decision-Making. http://knowledgecenter.csg.org/kc/system/files/SoundScience2014_FINAL_revision1.pdf (accessed April 13, 2018).

Courtney, H., J. Kirkland, and P. Viguerie. 1997. Strategy under uncertainty. *Harvard Business Review*. November–December 1997 Issue.

Funtowicz, S. 2006. *Interfaces between Science and Society*. Greenleaf Publications.

Haimes, Y.Y. 1998. *Risk modeling, assessment, and management*. New York: Wiley.

Haimes, Y.Y. 2004. *Risk modeling, assessment, and management*. Hoboken, NJ: John Wiley & Sons, 837 pp.

Henry, N.L. May–June 1974. Knowledge management: A new concern for public administration. *Public Administration Review* 34 (3): 189. DOI: 10.2307/974902.

Johnson, P. 2015. Avoiding decision paralysis in the face of uncertainty. *Harvard Business Review*. March 11, 2015. https://hbr.org/2015/03/avoiding-decision-paralysis-in-the-face-of-uncertainty.

Kahneman, D. 2011. *Thinking, fast and slow*. New York: Farrar, Straus and Giroux.

Keren, G. and K.H. Teigen. 2004. Yet another look at the heuristics and biases approach, entry. In D. Koehler and N. Harvey (eds.), *Blackwell handbook of judgment and decision making*, pp. 89–109. Malden, MA: Blackwell Publishing.

Kochenderfer, M.J. et al. 2015. *Decision making under uncertainty theory and application*. Cambridge, MA: MIT Press.

Lempert, R.J., S.W. Popper, and S.C. Bankes 2003. Shaping the next one hundred years: New methods for quantitative, long-term policy analysis. *Rand Corporation*. https://www.rand.org/content/dam/rand/pubs/monograph_reports/2007/MR1626.pdf.

Lipshitz, R. and O. Strauss 1997. Coping with uncertainty: A naturalistic decision-making analysis. *Organizational Behavior and Human Decision Processes* 69 (2): pp. 149–163.

Payne, J.W. and J.R. Bettman. 2004. Walking with the scarecrow: The information-processing approach to decision research, entry. In D. Koehler and N. Harvey (eds.), *Blackwell handbook of judgment and decision making*, pp. 110–132. Malden, MA: Blackwell Publishing.

Pfeiffer, J. 2012. *Interactive Decision Aids in e-Commerce*. Contributions to Management Science, DOI 10.1007/978-3-7908-2769-9 2, Berlin Heidelberg: Springer-Verlag.

Reeves, M. 2016. The world just got more uncertain and your strategy needs to adjust. *Harvard Business Review*. November 11, 2016. https://hbr.org/2016/11/the-world-just-got-more-uncertain-and-your-strategy-needs-to-adjust.

Riesch, H. 2013. Chapter 2 Levels of Uncertainty. In S. Roeser et al. (eds), *Essentials of Risk Theory*, Springer Briefs in Philosophy. DOI: 10.1007/978-94-007-5455-3_2.

Rowley, J. 2007. The wisdom hierarchy: Representations of the DIKW hierarchy. *Journal of Information and Communication Science* 33 (2): 163–180. DOI: 10.1177/0165551506070706.

Simon, H.A. 1955. A behavioral model of rational choice. *The Quarterly Journal of Economics* 69 (1): 99–118.

Simon, H.A. 1978. Rationality as process and product of thought. *American Economic Review* 68: 1–16.

Tversky, A. and D. Kahneman. 1974. Judgment under uncertainty: Heuristics and biases. *Science* New Series, 185 (4157). (Sep. 27, 1974): 1124–1131.

Vaes, K. 2013. *Understanding; Data, knowledge, information & wisdom.* https://kvaes. wordpress.com/2013/05/31/data-knowledge-information-wisdom (accessed July 17, 2018).

Van der Sluijs, J.P., M. Craye, S.O. Funtowicz, P. Kloprogge, J.R. Ravetz, and J.S. Risbey. 2005. Combining quantitative and qualitative measures of uncertainty in model based environmental assessment: The NUSAP System. *Risk Analysis* 25: 481–492.

Walker, W.E., R.J. Lempert, and J.H. Kwakkel. 2013. "Deep Uncertainty," entry. In Gass, S. and M. Fu (eds.), *Encyclopedia of operations research and management science*, 3rd ed. pp. 395–402. Springer.

Wardekker, A.J., J.P. van der Sluijs, P.H.M. Janssen, P. Kloprogge, and A.C. Petersen. 2008. Uncertainty communication in environmental assessments: Views from the Dutch science-policy interface. *Environmental Science & Policy* 11 (2008): 627–641.

Wikipedia. 2018a. *Adaption of the DIKW pyramid by US Army Knowledge Masters.* https://en.wikipedia.org/wiki/DIKW_pyramid (accessed July 17, 2018).

Wikipedia. 2018b. *DIKW pyramid* https://en.wikipedia.org/wiki/DIKW_pyramid (accessed October 27, 2017).

Yoe, C. 2017. *Principles of risk analysis for water resources.* U.S. Army Corps of Engineers, Institute for Water Resources.

# Index

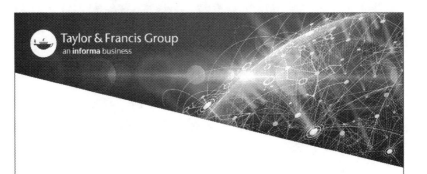

Printed in the United States
by Baker & Taylor Publisher Services